Body and Soul

Marie-Louise von Franz, Honorary Patron

**Studies in Jungian Psychology
by Jungian Analysts**

Daryl Sharp, General Editor

BODY AND SOUL

The Other Side
of Illness

Albert Kreinheder

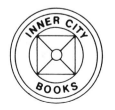

Canadian Cataloguing in Publication Data

Kreinheder, Albert, 1913-1990.
  Body and soul: the other side of illness

(Studies in Jungian psychology by Jungian analysts; 48)

ISBN 0-919123-49-X

1. Mind and body. 2. Soul.
3. Jung, C.G. (Carl Gustav), 1875-1961.
4. Kreinheder, Albert, 1913-1990.
5. Cancer—Patients—Biography.
I. Title. II. Series.

BF175.G37 1990   154   C90-094680-6

INNER CITY BOOKS
Box 1271, Station Q, Toronto, Canada M4T 2P4
Telephone (416) 927-0355
FAX 416-924-1814

Honorary Patron: Marie-Louise von Franz.
Publisher and General Editor: Daryl Sharp.
Senior Editor: Victoria Cowan.

INNER CITY BOOKS was founded in 1980 to promote the
understanding and practical application of the work of C.G. Jung.

Cover painting by Canadian artist Annie B. Knoop

Printed and bound in Canada

Contents

Foreword   7

1   The Day the Cat Died   11

2   Through Whose Eyes?   15

3   Weeding the Garden   19

4   Healing Is a Miracle   24

5   Living the Soul   28

6   Bring the Wheelchair   33

7   The Spirit Guide   36

8   Pains in the Chest   39

9   Where Is Passion Bred?   41

10   The Image Behind the Symptom   47

11   What If I Like the Way I Am?   51

12   There Is a Story   56

13   There Is a Power   59

14   More About the Power   63

15   Terror or Ecstasy?   65

16   Bleeding at the Mouth   71

17   Anxiety Can Kill   78

18   All Over the Skin   89

19   The Problem or the Power?   97

20   Why Not Change the Plot?   102

21   And After That the Dark   107

See final page for descriptions of other Inner City Books

Foreword

Healing of the mind, as well as healing of the body, probably was practiced in prehistoric times. In fact, it is quite probable that the earliest healing, except for cuts, bruises, broken bones and such, was to mend the soul or spirit of the afflicted one. When one's head split with pain or one's belly burned from an inner fire, what else could be amiss?

In more recent times, shamans, witch doctors and, most recently, even psychotherapists, with the backing of the science of psychology, have offered their services in the treatment of bodily ills. With the advent of science, shamans became psychologists and witch doctors became physicians and seldom the twain shall meet. Until Sigmund Freud and C.G. Jung.

Freud envisioned in psychosomatic cases a body victimized by unredeemed complexes fostered by botched toilet training; Jung took somewhat the same view, but substituted perverse archetypes for parental "abuse." Going one step further, though not the first to do so, Dr. Albert Kreinheder imagined an intertwining or intermingling of body and mind rather than a simple cause and effect relationship. What makes his book original is that it presents a theoretic concept (not the term he would have used) and a method of treatment based upon his own immediate experience and founded upon extensive scientific training and a lengthy personal analysis.

But what makes his work truly unique is that amazingly, in this day of published jargonistic psychobabble passing for science, Kreinheder has written a supremely readable book (many chapters read like prose poetry) about the body and the psyche without it being "psychological." He understood that the essence of human experience is not psychological and rational; it is something ineffable and immediate, passionate and painful, spiritual and profane, that must be both endured and celebrated. Kreinheder's psychology stems from *his* life and *his* approaching death. And, as noted above, it is founded upon a sound scientific education.

Nor is this book narrowly about himself. When Kreinheder writes, "Everything in heaven and earth affects me and is affected by me," he is echoing Walt Whitman's "Song of Myself," which he knew quite well. That is, he uses the personal pronouns I and we to mean Everyman.

The personal Albert Kreinheder was born in 1913 in Buffalo, New York. He attended Syracuse University and earned a B.A. and M.A. in English. His intention at the time was to support a career of writing with teaching, but World War Two interrupted his plans. A pacifist, he spent the war in conscientious objector camps working in national forests. At war's end, he enrolled at the Claremont Graduate School in Claremont, California, as a doctoral student in clinical psychology. With the award of a Ph.D. in 1952, he entered private practice in Los Angeles. A little over ten years later he became a Jungian analyst through the C.G. Jung Institute of Los Angeles. At different times he served the Institute as Director of Training, Chairman of the Certifying Board and President.

About fifteen years ago, Kreinheder, an athlete in his youth and a jogger before jogging shoes were invented, was made virtually immobile by arthritis. Though he tried a combination of medical, nutritional and chiropractic treatment, it was by an intensive exploration through active imagination into the reason for the pain that he achieved a full remission. The consequence of his healing experience was a series of articles in the Los Angeles Jungian journal *Psychological Perspectives* and lec-

how, through active imagination, he had been healed.

Two and a half years before he started writing *Body and Soul,* he underwent surgery in which cancerous tissue was discovered and removed. The first chapter of this book is about that experience. In succeeding chapters he tells of his way of confronting the specter of pain and death both in his own instance and in the cases of several patients. The book was finished weeks before his seventy-sixth birthday. Four months later, in April 1990, *Body and Soul* was accepted for publication; in less than two months he died of a reoccurrence of the cancer.

This book is a last testament of a dying man, a man with profound insight—but it is about life and living. The last chapter is Kreinheder's gift to his readers. He tells us all how to die with dignity, equanimity and courage. That is the way he died.

Kreinheder may have been familiar with the lyrics of the popular song of the thirties from which he borrowed the title of his book. Three lines from it could be his address to Death:

> *My life a hell you're making,*
> *You know I'm yours for just the taking,*
> *I gladly surrender my life to you, body and soul.*

"Healing may take place in death," his spirit medium said. "Death is the final healing."

*

Al Kreinheder asked that his book be dedicated to the loving partner of his last eleven years, Linda Gilbert, and to the spiritual inspiration of his healing, his friend, colleague and mentor, Dr. Kieffer Frantz.

William O. Walcott, Ph.D.,
Jungian Analyst, Los Angeles

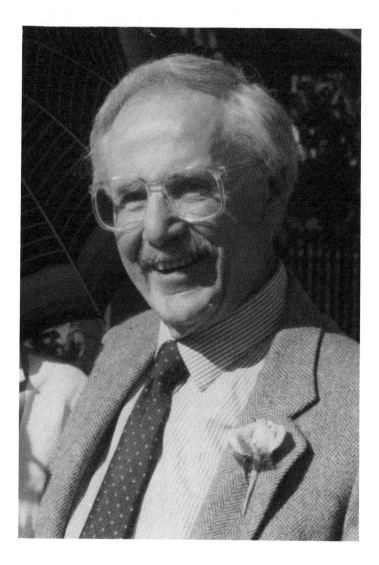

1

The Day the Cat Died

The story begins with Willie, and Willie is a cat. He's grey like a dark cloud and tiger striped. He loves me. In a non-complicated, matter-of-fact way, like "Of course I love you. Whoever thought differently?" But that's all past tense now.

He was part of the family. There was Linda (my wife), Michael (stepson, age 10), myself and Willie. We were his pride of lions. He lay on the bed with us, our television-watching bed. Purr. Purr. Or he walked over us at his pleasure.

I also have a wider community, though pretty narrowed now because of this age thing. The doctors are part of it, my personal HMO. They monitor my body month by month and tell me how to take care of it. There was a small growth at the groin, probably a fatty cyst, said Dr. Mosky. "Nothing at all really, but let's get it out and see for sure."

They got me onto my back in the hospital, and Dr. Kukenbecker, the surgeon, was digging into my groin. Why was it taking so long? Slowly, carefully, bit by bit. Then into a bottle and down to the lab. He was still sewing me up when the lab report came back.

It was melanoma, he said—in a monotone, as if he was reciting the rosary. I knew what melanoma was, but not exactly at that moment. Not until the next day did I recall that melanoma was cancer, and a very serious kind, especially when it has advanced to the lymph node. That was the situation—melanoma, lymph node, left groin.

It was necessary, Dr. K. said, to find the origin, the pri-

11

mary site. It starts somewhere and then advances to the lymph node. Nothing was visible on the skin surfaces, so a real operation was in order. Exploratory surgery. A six-inch incision linking up with my old hernia scar, going into the peritoneum to the deeper arteries and lymph nodes, the whole pelvic landscape.

Dr. Kukenbecker is six feet three and weighs 240 pounds. He inspires both confidence and fear. Anyone that substantial must be twice as mature and sensible as I am. But how can he probe delicately with those big fingers into the most sensitive cavity of my body?

I had a community—Dr. Mosky, Dr. Harwitt, Dr. Klein and Dr. Kukenbecker. And also Linda and Michael and Willie. Dear Willie, I loved him so. He was like God himself, his paws on my face, licking my hands, clawing me playfully.

Two hours after the big surgical event I was lying on the hospital bed, still splattered and stunned by the six-inch hole in my belly. The phone rang, and reaching for it, I felt as if my groin was splitting open all over again.

"We've got a family problem." It was Linda. "Willie's dead," she said. "The lady next door found him and came over sobbing." She had just lost her husband a month ago, and now this.

"I buried him," Linda said, "got a shovel out of the garage and buried him. And now Michael's crying, wants me to dig Willie up so he can hold him. I don't know what to do. I found Michael covered with dirt, clawing the ground, trying to find Willie."

Well, she had to dig him up anyway because the Animal Control people told her that it's against the law to bury animals. "Put him in a plastic bag out on the curb, and we'll pick him up." So she put him at the curb in a black bag with a big paper label that said, "Dead Cat."

While she was telling me all this, Dr.Kukenbecker came into my hospital room. Always the same tone. Good news, bad news, just the facts. "There's nothing back there" (in the pelvic cavity), he said. "It's all normal. And your arteries look good too, no arteriosclerosis. You can go home this afternoon."

I no longer see life as strictly rational, and I am coming to believe that many of life's events are fated, happening according to the dream of some whimsical god. It was not strange therefore for me to murmur to myself, "Oh my God, here I am alive, and Willie's dead." And further: "I'm alive because Willie's dead. He died so I could live."

Somebody in the community had to go, and Willie was chosen. He was the greatest soul of all of us. There's not a great deal that Willie was able to do. Even though he always seemed like God incarnate with infinite instinctual wisdom, he didn't have much clout in a purely practical sense. But he did spread an ambiance of contentment over the whole family. And he knew how to die. I'm alive because he's dead. That's the way I understand it. That is my perception, and my perceptions are what I live by.

We are moving into a new house, and Michael has requested a Willie-colored carpet for his bedroom.

I do feel now that it is really something special for me to be alive. Perhaps I'm still here because of some important thing I need to do. Just what I don't know. But my not knowing has no trace of doubt or confusion.

Perhaps it is to do this writing. Writing is difficult, yet it has become for me a way to emotional health. In that deep concentration with the computer screen before my face, I am drawn into another world. I am myself in a more special way, straining only to be myself in as pure a form as possible. It is another reality, a reality where I feel whole and new again. As long as I go on writing, I believe that I shall keep on living. But if I stop, if I lose connection to that healing reality, I fear my days will be numbered.

2
Through Whose Eyes?

I sent a copy of the Willie story to Dr. K. since he was one of the principal actors in the drama. But I never heard from him. When I saw him later for post-op checkups, he didn't mention the story. Nor did I. No doubt he regarded me as a sentimental dreamer, made even more spacey than usual by having my body cut open, not to mention that big word, cancer, now being in me and on me like a new middle name.

I read the story again. And I rethought it. I could see his point of view. In a way I'm glad he has this cold-blooded, factual attitude. What's real is real, and if you can't touch it or smell it, it's not really real. I don't want him fainting on me when his big fingers are groping through my torso.

The Willie story, as I put it together, is like a child's wishful fantasy. This goes with this, and that goes with that because I like it to. When I am pre-logical, anything goes with anything, just as I wish it. The pre-conscious part of ourselves reasons like that. And if the body were to reason, which it probably does, it would be in this primitive, dreamlike kind of logic. It is almost as if the body were always communicating, expressing and manifesting itself in various ways. As if the body itself were sentient, feeling, emotive, highly eloquent, but in a totally non-verbal and non-linear way.

If we could learn again to "be" our body selves, then its animalistic, childlike, instinctive knowingness would be there side by side with the Dr. Kukenbecker self. When I think of Willie, and I let myself go with the charmed illogic of the Willie story, then I am with my body and not fighting it. Then I feel

15

alive and I feel well. It awakens a different state of consciousness. And for me that particular kind of consciousness is with
me in my writing. It is the thing sought, the "thing" I am going
to talk more and more about in various ways in the ensuing
chapters. That thing, that attitude, that world of different consciousness, is the psychic climate where healing takes place. It
is the place of soul stuff. It is that something which we are all
seeking and wishing for without even knowing what we want
or need.

Doctors who cut people open have to believe in the reality
of the flesh and the blade and the one-to-one relationship of
virus to blood to cell to lymph node. Dr. K. might become
paralyzed with self-doubt if I got him believing in the Willie
story.

But we patients need our fantasies and our dreams and our
mythologies. Let him see it his way. His way has respectabil-
ity, and it even works well most of the time for most things.
The whole world out there can't be totally wrong. But let me
also see it my way. My way is not a delusion. It is my experience, my reality, my psychological truth. And it makes me
well. I could have been dead three times in the last ten years if I
didn't have this "psychological reality" to pull me through.

Why is their reality any better than mine? What is reality
anyway? That limited, rigid, objectively-evident view of reality
probably caused the sickness in the first place. The effort it
takes. The tension. Always conforming and repressing and
holding our behavior with effort to that hypothetical norm that
has become the agreed-upon standard of sanity.

I know when I am up against forces bigger than myself.
Events unfold, and we adapt to them. That's how it works. I
trust science, as far as it goes. So I do what logic and common
sense and the best-informed research suggests, and then be-

yond that is something, something strange and unbelievable. She, It, They, the Things, the Influences. Are they watching me? Am I at the center of some purpose, some meaning?

It seems that there are two realities. There is a kind of inner or separate reality that screens events through our imagination and fantasy and by which we perceive entirely different connections and meanings. These are beyond the scope of fact and sense but are nevertheless very influential in forming our behavior and especially our bodily reactions.

Though this side of things seems irrelevant and crazy to most people, it is a part of being human. If you can let yourself be crazy without losing your sanity, there is a comfort and perhaps a wisdom. There was for me a healthier health than I ever had before. The migraine headaches went away, and the stiff necks, and now my joints hang looser and I sleep at night.

As Ann Landers says, "A little craziness now and then could save you from permanent brain damage." *(Los Angeles Times,* June 4, 1989)

Of course, there's more to it than just cultivating the art of being crazy. But that's an important step along the way. To flow with what comes, to welcome everything that you are. Those bizarre impulses, those fantastic thoughts, to accept what is without first questioning whether it is approved.

If you listen to enough research reports, as I have, you sometimes begin to wonder why they do these studies at all. Often they find out nothing for sure, or they discover after diligent fact-gathering and astonishing statistical feats that there is, for instance, a correlation of .73 between coffee drinking and staying awake.

Truth is truly elusive, and your truth is not my truth. And down the line in a few years what we had full scientific proof for may turn out no longer to be true at all. Yet somewhere in this maze of eager scientific publication there emerges occasionally a true "truth" that changes the whole direction of civilization. But the great illuminators who fathered these significant bursts of knowledge were noted not so much for their drudge work as for their astonishing hypotheses.

It is important to test and prove a hypothesis, but the true brilliance is in the brain that conceived the hypothesis. Hypotheses arise out of the interaction of fact and imagination. New truths are discovered by people who have the imagination to see them. Then scientific experimentation is necessary to verify their insights.

3
Weeding the Garden

The big C is a big thing, and I didn't blithely think that it was suddenly all better now just because the cat died. The cat helped out and saved me from immediate danger, but there were still fears and doubts and worries. It's hard suddenly to feel like a pure child of God right after they've dug a melanoma out of you. Undoubtedly there remained some cleaning up to do and some changes to be made. And, as a matter of fact, several years later there was a recurrence of the melanoma.

I had a dream about Dr. Kukenbecker. The Dr. K. of my dreams is not the same as the other Dr. K. I respect them both, but the dream Dr. K. is rounded out with the qualities of the archetypal healer and the wise old man.

In the dream he took me from my old house into a new house. Then he began to remove weeds from around the house. These weeds were that pesky stuff we call devil's grass that seems to come up again and again and spread all over the place no matter how many of the roots you get out.

I've seen devil's grass wipe out flower beds and very quickly take command of a whole landscaping job. It is the cancer of the garden, with virulent tentacles grabbing a new foothold inch by inch. I was in a new house now, a fresh attitude perhaps, and that was promising. Dr. K. was still with me, patiently removing the "little stranglers," not unlike the way he had dug out every little piece from my groin. He needed my help, as if I couldn't just stand by passively and hope to get well.

Continuing the dream in my imagination, I asked him how

19

I could help. And Dr. K., the dream Dr. K., responded:

"Be robust in your health so that your healthy growth will overcome and crowd out the intruder. Also make efforts to uproot and destroy the evil enemy."

I asked him how I could do that. He replied:

"Think. The answer is in you. We are dealing with death, with the destroyer. It is the evil encroacher. It is the venom, the poison, the evil. It is all the twisted, dark, malevolent, vengeful, crooked and hateful feelings. It is also the bitter, heavy, defeatist sense that all is lost, that it's all over. It is the viper, the octopus, the tentacles that are ready to grip you into submission. Be aware of all those dark feelings, but don't give into them. Ask for help from the great benevolent power. Feel the energy of triumph and ascendance. Be with the healing power. Perceive it. Embrace it. Let it live in you. Turn also to your dreams. Find the hope that is in your dreams. There is the fullness. There is the hope that balances the despair, the life energy that will counterbalance the death energy. There is no sense in dying before your time. The parabola of your life reaches on to the future. Do not cut it short."

Four days later I had another dream.

I was attending a professional meeting. Dr. Gallup was presenting a paper on the progress of an illness. His paper was about a woman who had been told that she must have an operation. Her story was illustrated in a book which had pictures showing her talking to relatives, leaving to go to the hospital, talking to the doctor, taking leave of her lover, etc. There was also a series of poems in which she expressed her feelings. Then in another scene it was a rainy, dreary day. I was with several of my professional colleagues, leaders in their local societies. We see coming toward us out of the ocean a procession of elephants.

Dr. Gallup was an M.D., now deceased, who was on the Certifying Board which examined me in my final oral examination before I became a Jungian analyst. His presence in the dream therefore recalls an important initiatory experience, and gives an impression that a further initiation is now taking place. The initiation is not of my conscious ego self into a new professional role, but now it is an initiation of the inner feminine, of the anima. The anima is generally thought to be the soul image in a man's unconscious. We may conclude, then, that the soul has been sick, and that my body in its illness is reflecting that sickness of my deeper soul.

We can also acknowledge that a process of healing is underway, and that it includes some fairly radical procedures, i.e., going to the hospital, going to a foreign country, taking leave of her relatives and even of her lover. We may assume also that it is an initiation, entailing for her an entry into a level of greater importance.

Since the woman in the dream had written poems, I felt a responsibility to record them, literally to become an instrument through which her poetic feelings could be made manifest. So in as free a way as possible, I let her use my hand and my words to give visible shape to her longings and to the despair within her. Here is one of her poems:

> *How can I cry*
> *when no one hears my cry?*
> *How can I weep*
> *when tears have left me dry?*
> *How can I see when darkness clouds my eye?*
> *Come blessed friend and find me*
> *you and I.*

And here is another, expressing her feelings as she entered the hospital for her surgery and for whatever other things were to happen to her:

> *Will I see the daylight dawning*
> *after this long night of longing?*
> *Will a vision come to wake me*
> *out of death to life hereafter?*
> *Save me someone from the darkness.*
> *Shine a light so I may see.*

One might ask why I think I know the interpretations to my own dreams. Can't a single dream be seen in a lot of different ways? Yes, of course, it is true that there are many possible interpretations, each perhaps just as plausible. However, the dream is my dream and it has come to me for my benefit. Therefore the correct meaning for me is the meaning that sinks in, that changes my consciousness and my behavior. Moreover, much of what I have done with the dreams is not interpretation at all, but is an amplifying and enriching of the experience by the use of imagination.

I became more aware of how I had neglected the anima and had lived most predominantly out of my masculine side. Before, if I noticed her at all, it was to see her merely as an amusement, stimulating my sexual desire, being charming and provocative. Now she seems ready to come into her maturity, to carry the soul function, guiding me and inspiring me toward union with the divine.

The transformation she was about to undergo seemed to me to be one that would orient her more strongly to the Self, thinking of the Self as the center of the psyche, the place of immense power where the ego and the unconscious, the sacred and the profane, meet and unite.

I felt that the parade of elephants coming forth out of the sea was the advent into consciousness of the Self. Along with the image of the elephants, I heard the song, "When the saints come marching in." Recollecting the image of those powerful beasts swaying majestically as they march toward me gives me a feeling of strength, of victory, of invincible power. I feel within myself the energy of health, of a wholeness that can overcome all those "little stranglers."

4
Healing Is a Miracle

So the cat died, and the cancer went away, and it hasn't come back. Not yet at least. And I feel as if I am living in a state of childlike wonder. I like it that way. It feels good. There is no tension, and I don't feel sick at all. I am the child I used to be. I've sloughed off a lot of responsibility. The world goes on somehow without my directing it. The air caresses me, and my energy expands into my surroundings.

It's all because I became a child again. To think like a child, to move like a child, to believe like a child. Recently I cut my finger. It was bleeding and stinging with pain, but now one week later it is all new again. Healing is a miracle. Life itself is a miracle, the rose emerging from seed and bud, the cocoon giving forth a butterfly.

For healing we must think miracle. Everything in heaven and earth affects me and is affected by me. When we stand apart and look at life, analyzing it, separating it into discrete pieces, we cut ourselves off from life and we damage a vital link in the chain of being. From our detached viewpoint we conclude that A causes B, and we think we understand. We think we have knowledge. But this kind of understanding is actually the beginning of chaos because it is a false knowledge that makes us feel superior to the rose and superior to the butterfly. In our sophistication we have lost the fundamental basis of wisdom. We have lost the attitude of wonder. And we have lost an appreciation of the miracle of life.

Somehow we feel safer if we can think the world into a rational mechanical mold. Then we no longer gasp with awe at

24

the wonders surrounding us. That's the split. Humdrum, plodding, stepwise, a cautious mind with tunnel vision, sadly unrelated to the infinite riches all around. When the consciousness is dead and lifeless, afraid of imagination, afraid of impulse, afraid of instinct, then these closed attitudes restrict the body and also hinder the healing process.

Sickness, when it comes, impresses one with the inevitability of death. Then comes a vision of one's own lifeless body. Contemplating the inert deadness of death makes us realize that in us and around us on every side is this astonishing miracle of life. How beautiful the world is! How wistfully we realize that soon we will no longer enjoy these wonders, and the life spirit will be gone from the body forever.

So it is that sickness and the accompanying thoughts of death may expand our mood toward the larger universe and deemphasize everyday concerns. By awakening us to the reality of the sacred dimension, sickness acts to promote salvation and the healing of the soul.

Ordinarily our consciousness is limited, full of facts and things, walled off from the full miracle and the full splendor of life and therefore not closely in tune with the healing power.

That "other world" which we call the archetypal or the sacred dimension seems to be wholly other than our personal ego self. It is not "part of me" or "my unconscious." It is *the* unconscious. It is non-personal or supra-personal. When we confront it, when it touches us, we feel ourselves to be in the presence of the divine. We are surprised, frightened, awed, as if we have met something uncanny and miraculous. I felt that way when Willie died, as if my life had been touched by the hand of fate.

It is this event, the meeting of the human and the divine, that makes miracle cures possible. It is not enough to have the healing energy in you. It is always there. But it is very important to actually perceive its physical presence.

Unless the conscious meeting takes place, the healing process does not reach its full potential. We are reminded of Faust to whom the spirits said, "We were always here, but you did not see us." Or of Jesus who lamented, "I came among you, but you knew me not."

Plato has said that whenever anyone has an experience of original beauty (an archetypal experience), it causes the feathers to sprout. As he explained, in the olden days the soul was known to be feathered, and the goose bumps that arise on the skin are the sprouting of the feathers of the soul.

Even today, whenever we cross paths with some presence from that other world, we feel a chill, a warmth, a creeping of the flesh, as the feathers begin to sprout.

When the archetypal energies touch our awareness, it is a meeting of the sacred and the profane. And it is both a psychic and a physical experience, not just in the mind, but also with definite feather-sprouting sensations in the body. These bodily sensations may at first be somewhat disturbing, but as one grows more trusting of the "totally other," they can become positively ecstatic.

A stream of fire runs through the body, healing the ills in every area it enters. It is like an instant surge of health. It is a momentary union of body and soul. When it happens, you feel whole, at one, and healed of your ills. Ideally this meeting of sacred and profane happens on a daily basis. However, it is not accomplished by perfunctory rituals, not by faithful journal writing, not by daily meditation nor rote prayers to the Virgin Mary (though such things may help, who knows?). All we understand is that when it happens, we know. Because then the feathers sprout. There is beauty, and there is truth. "That is all ye know and all ye need to know."

When the opposites touch, a tremendous energy is released. Miracles of healing are then possible, and astonishing disturbances, both good and bad, will then occur. So however effective and necessary the traditional remedies may be, such as rest and diet and care and medication, there is no intervention with effects as dramatic as what may happen when mind meets body, when ego meets archetype, to create soul.

5
Living the Soul

Did you ever think to ask yourself, "Who am I? Just who am I anyway?" It seems on the one hand to be the simplest question in the world. And on the other hand, as in the admonition to "Know thyself," it contains all the mysteries of human meaning.

There must be more to me, I tell myself, than what I appear to be from the outside. I am a psychologist with certain professional attainments. I am a man who has a wife and some grown children. I have a biography and a genealogy. Probably two double-spaced pages would suffice to give an adequate account of my outer look. You might call me an introvert and an intuitive-feeling kind of person, with a body that's half athlete and half bookworm. I've written some articles and given some lectures and I was on the swim team in college. Et cetera. Anyway, it's no big deal. All the information that anyone would care to know about me could still be covered in two pages, double spaced.

One day one of my students, someone studying to become an analyst, asked me what I was working at, what was my specialty, my interest, my thing. And that was almost as hard to answer as the question about who I am. All of a sudden I felt like a failure. Maybe I should be giving seminars on witchcraft or writing papers on the inner life of Edgar Allen Poe. But no, I didn't seem to have any special thing. I was just here. Why am I not discovering the dreambody like Arnold Mindell, or the ego-self axis like Ed Edinger, or telling about the mind-body connection like Ernest Rossi? I wondered, am I supposed to make some big contribution like that, or would it be sufficient just to say, "I am. Lo, I am alive"?

It is peculiar. It's as if I'm deliberately not doing anything because I don't want to get messed up with that crazy, ravenous beast part of myself that thirsts for some kind of position or glory. Yet I ought to do something. I've got to realize myself, be somebody. And then there is an answering voice: "Well, you are somebody."

Then if I am somebody, I suppose it will come forth and show itself in action. There is no essential difference between the being and the doing. The "me" wants to come forth and be what it is possible to be. It's not megalomania. It's just that I want to say, "Please World, see what I am. Isn't it wonderful what I am? Isn't everyone wonderful if only we knew them?" I want to know myself, so that everyone else can know me, and I can bring forth all that's stirring inside of me. No, it's not big. Just average. Einstein was average. Shakespeare was average. Marilyn Monroe was average.

Human beings are by nature astonishingly wonderful, just in their average state as human beings. Sometimes with certain people the wonder shows through and it is evident to everyone. We see clearly the very fine thing a human being is capable of being—an Einstein, a Shakespeare, a Marilyn Monroe.

If only we knew ourselves! This quest for self is the yearning for soul. It is the archetypal yearning to become again as a child. Being a child is so very important because—as it seems to me now in retrospect—when I was a child, I was my true self, living my own soul. As an adult, on the other hand, too often I was acting out performances that bore little resemblance to what I really was. And that caused so much tension and so much wear and tear on the body that it has seemed to me to be extremely important to seek out the soul and to get so acquainted with it that I would be living it every day in my behavior and feeling it in my body.

The soul lives on the very edge of miracle. When I find my soul, even if it happens just for a moment and only once in a while, I feel right then as if a miracle has occurred. The soul is the part of me that is most truly myself. And it is also, I would say, the part of every person that is most truly similar to the image of God. So, if that is true, the experience of soul is also the experience of God, as if our soul-self touches and coalesces with God. That is a tremendously big idea: The soul-self is where the human and the divine meet and affect each other. Furthermore, if we are there, if we live on the plane of soul, then we are as sound and healthy, both physically and emotionally, as it is possible for a human being to be.

Yet in practice for the most part we all live like imposters, hiding our true selves. We are aliens in a strange land, troubled and confused, just not quite the way we think we ought to be. And since we don't at all understand what is missing, we have the pathetic hope that the gap will be filled by a better job, a classier car, or the right partner in love. This aching discontent has been called loss of soul. Without even knowing it, we are frantically seeking our soul, that missing ingredient that is going to complete us and make life wonderful at last. If all else fails, maybe we will win the lottery. We long for a miracle, for a shiny new self. There must be something there, an inkling of a real possibility, or why would we continue to crave it? There is something within us that we project outward, but it is not really to be found outward because it is ourselves that we seek.

For 20 years I wanted to have a Cadillac. Now I have a Cadillac, but it doesn't do it. Somehow the soul went out of the Cadillac. I always wanted a house with a view. Now I have a house with a view. I can see the ocean, but the soul went out of the house too. If you've seen one ocean, you've seen them all. I wanted a woman with long legs who liked sex. And, believe it or not, I found her. She used to be my long lost soul, but the soul went out of her too. And then I started looking at mysterious women with misty eyes who wrote poetry. Women like this were harder to find, but they do exist, and the one I found captured my soul for 23 weeks. Then disillusionment set in.

So I have started to see myself as two different people. There is the empirical me that is described by all these external things I am. And then there is what I call my soul-self. There are times when I can say to myself, "This is the real me. Now I am really myself." And there is at these moments a great feeling of well-being, of fullness and joy. I seem then to expand beyond my ordinary self, as if the soul includes not only me but also powers beyond me. It is a larger self, much larger than my own person, but somehow fully me also.

It is not easy to describe. But I felt it that day at age 11 when I got the bicycle. I always wanted a bicycle. Nothing was more important than that I should have a bicycle. I could not possibly ever grow tired of riding a bicycle. That would always be a delight, and I would never again be bored. There were times on that bicycle that every facet of myself was absorbed in the joyous experience of me and the bicycle and the wind in my face. It didn't last forever, of course, but while it did, it was glorious.

Another time I was hiking in the forest, smelling the hemlock and the dark scent of decaying leaves, feeling the effort in my leg muscles. "This is it," I thought. "This is what I must do. Now I am where I should be."

When my soul is touched, I know what I'm here for. My whole purpose and destiny is just to be. Just the sense of being that soul that I am. That does it. That is absolutely enough.

I guess a person would never even have an inkling of the soul if everything always went smoothly in the ego life. It is actually through our ego defeats that we discover the opportunity for living the soul. We have to experience the utter humiliation and failure of our ego mania before we can even know that something is missing. There is disillusion after disillusion because everything "out there" is ultimately disappointing. Only God is God. And only the soul is the soul.

If "soul" seems to be too cloudy a concept or too poetic, let's prefer to keep it that way. To know thyself is as impossible as knowing God. Let's not lose the mystery by pretending to a knowledge that we do not have. All we can do is talk around the word soul—amplify it, illustrate it, give anecdotes and analogies. When you find it, you will know.

If you find it and stay with it, you will be healed. The philosopher Plotinus has said that in sickness the body has lost contact with the soul and no longer resembles it. Living the soul means that our activities, our thoughts, the total unfolding of our life's journey is a living out of the soul's meanings and intentions.

For the last few weeks I have been watching an amaryllis bulb push up from the earth and form itself into this astonishing crimson creation. There are, I know, scientific explanations of how such things can be. But I say spare me your explanations. Let me be a crazy, soft-brained romantic. That seems more substantial than those wisely contrived scientific accounts. The awe, the mystery, the unknowing are also part of the event, and it would be (shall we say unscientific?) to leave them out.

6
Bring the Wheelchair

Before I got cancer, I had several other serious diseases, namely arthritis and tuberculosis. It is important to recount my experiences with these diseases because they furnish further understanding of the meaning of illness and of the possibilities for healing.

I thought I was ready for the wheelchair and that life as I knew it was over. It had been building up over the months. The pain and the stiffness and the debility. This was happening about ten years ago. First my hip and then my knee, then elbows and ankles and fingers and toes. Even the jaw bones. Rheumatoid arthritis, a strange invasive disease, had taken command of my body. And my mind also, because I was questioning the meaning of everything and why I was here, feeling cloudy and unrelated, not sure what things were real or important. When you are aware all the time of your body, with its pain and its fatigue determining everything you do, there is a big realignment of priorities, and nothing is quite the same as it was before. Life itself seems very tenuous, and that shifts one's perspective tremendously.

Especially if you are not sure if you will ever walk again. One afternoon I lay down for a sun bath and, like a turtle turned over on its back, I couldn't get back up. I had to crawl to the steps and worm my way up step by step. Sometimes fear overcame me, especially since I lived alone, watching my muscles atrophying from lack of use, wondering if one day my joints would be locked so tightly that I could not even pull myself to the refrigerator.

33

The body was weakened, and the mind dimmed. I would get up in the morning, throw a breakfast together, shuffle through some papers, and two hours later I would be back in bed again exhausted.

Yet strangely, in spite of all this and even with the pain, there was also at times a rich feeling of pleasure and a charming sense of indulgence in being sick. The world with its responsibilities faded into unreality. And a different consciousness arose, as if with a weaker ego the unconscious leaked through and thereby brought about a closer meeting of the sacred and the profane.

Sometimes I wanted just to drift and to imagine that I could hear the hum of the grass growing. It was like the purring of a cat. Everything around me, the trees, the plants, the earth, the air, were softly vibrating like the purring of a cat.

I was taking 24 aspirins a day. The dry bones were grating against each other and the pain was awesome. I began to wonder who was choreographing my life. I certainly wasn't. And that was a lesson right there. It was something I had suspected before and had learned theoretically, but which had never really sunk in. Because only now did I know for sure that whoever was determining my fate was not I.

Neither I nor the whole medical establishment as my paid deputies had any power to modify this situation that was dominating my life. It was a humbling experience. I had felt inferior before but never humbled, never in this particular existential way.

It was the pain. The pain was bigger than I, stronger than I. It had more authority over me than I had over myself.

I thought of the pain as my adversary, as my master. One night when I felt that I could stand it no longer, I spoke to the pain:

ME: You hold me tight in your grip and do not let me go. If you crave my undivided attention, you have received it. Whatever I attend to, I must also attend to you. Even as I write, I feel you in my hand and in all parts of my body. I am terribly frightened of you. Why? Why are you here?

PAIN: I am here to get your attention. I make known my presence. I have a power beyond your power. My will surpasses yours. You cannot prevail over me, but I can easily prevail over you.

ME: But why must you show me this power and destroy me with it?

PAIN: I show you because I will no longer let you disregard me. You can no longer treat me as if I am not. You will know my power, and you will humble yourself before me. I am the first of all things, and all things spring from me, and without me there is nothing. I want you to see me and feel me and hear me and to bring to me the best of yourself. I want to be closely in touch with you in your thoughts at all times. Now, with my presence in you, you can no longer live the same old way. You cannot use your mind in the old ways, for now you must give yourself only to contemplation of me. And out of this will come many good things.

This was the beginning of many dialogues with the pain god. It was the beginning of a different perception of the pain. I felt the pain now to be a presence, an intelligence, an entity, an extremely powerful demon who was intimately involved with me. The pain was still painful, but it was also a companion, a companion who, though he chastened me, also loved me deeply. . .

7

The Spirit Guide

Much of the knowledge I have about healing came to me from my "spirit guide." When I was 64 years old, I dreamed of a deceased colleague, Dr. Kieffer Frantz. In the dream he had woven a coat for me. It was loose fitting in somewhat of a Mexican style and had patterns of bright color.

It reminded me of Joseph's coat of many colors, and I began to believe that in some small way my myth—my story or my meaning—was similar to that of Joseph. Dr. Frantz had been like a father to me, and I felt that with the gift of the coat he was calling upon me to continue his unfinished work. Dr. Frantz had a deep dedication to "soul work," and he was particularly interested in the unity of the body and the psyche. He had been the director for many years of the C.G. Jung Clinic of Los Angeles. He was highly regarded because of his integrity and his devotion to the highest standards in his teaching and in his work with patients. A few months before his death he had resigned his position at the Clinic in order to give more emphasis to his healing researches and to his own soul journey.

I began to write dialogues in which Dr. Frantz and I spoke to each other. After about 35 of such dialogues, and when I was very close to the exact age at which he was when he died, our talks turned to the subject of healing. Without the benefit of these dialogues with Dr.Frantz I could not have generated out of myself the same understanding of healing that I now have. When I am in my dialogues with him, I fully imagine that I am addressing his spirit, and I am very thankful that I possess the gift of belief that enables me to do so.

The philosophy of illness and healing that I received from Dr. Frantz was transparently simple. Illness represented a break in our wholeness, a disturbance in the man-universe relationship. Man's position in the universe is one of delicate balance. Each individual is unique but is also connected in some way to all the rest of the universe.

As Kieffer put it, "When I died and came over to this side, I suddenly experienced wholeness in a way that no mortal ever knows it. I was immersed in wholeness. The universe flowed through me as if in a moment I was all. I knew all.

"Now," he said, "being in this place, I am completely well. And being so, at last I know the nature of health. Every illness is an onslaught upon us as we are. Somehow we get so alienated from the whole of life that a very extreme invasion is necessary to break in upon the hardened formation of oneself. We must be weakened and crushed so that we will finally be so loosened and liquified that the life spirit can flow into us again. To be sick is to be shut off, to be isolated. Every disease is like an invading force trying to destroy our rigid forms and make us more whole.

"With every invading symptom there comes also a symbolic content, and it is the task of the soul to expand itself so it can include the invading images and symbols. This may be a struggle, but ultimately it is not a struggle but an expansive, releasing process as we grow beyond our former boundaries."

"But," I asked him, "what specifically can I do—if I have stiff joints or sinus allergies or pains in my chest? It doesn't seem enough just to accept it. It seems more natural to strengthen my defense and get rid of it."

"Yes," he replied, "but that's still your old self talking. The disease won't let us live the same old way. It actually comes to destroy the way we are. The blockages in your respiratory tract, the stiffness in your movement—these are because of the way you have held yourself. They are from a guarded, fearful, cautious posture, a carefulness to control tears and anger and free spontaneous movements. The symptoms are the crying out of the body, telling you it has had enough. The symptoms will tear you apart at the very places where you have held too tightly."

"Yes," I agreed. "They attack me at the place of my defense. They break through my armor. But I cannot automatically let everything flow in and out. It's more than I can cope with."

"It may seem so," he said, "but not really. We never get more than we can handle. Even if it means death, death can be handled. The object of healing is not to stay alive. It is to move closer to wholeness. Healing may take place in death, death as the final healing. Whatever comes to us is ours, and we can handle it."

8
Pains in the Chest

It seems to me that much of one's life history and the history of one's family background is written into the twisted shapes and infirmities of the body. My old chest pains were returning, the aching stitch in the side that dated from the time I had pleurisy at age 15. The chest pain awakened all the worries that I too, like my mother before me, would get tuberculosis and I too would die. And sure enough, along with the rheumatoid arthritis and all my related debilities, there was additional damage. The sputum analysis revealed that I had active tuberculosis.

I became aware that I had an unconscious identification with my mother, mostly having to do with my body, that my body was like her body or even that it was her body. Or my body actually was my mother. Then it seemed also that it was not just my mother but was the great mother goddess herself. And I had the chest pain and all my other ailments because I was on very bad terms with her. I spoke to her, to the mother goddess, and she told me that she expected to be loved and worshiped by me.

So I learned to pray to the mother goddess, to worship and adore her. This was a great accomplishment for me because I had always been an anti-mother person. When I was training to be a Jungian analyst and was trying to convince my mentors what good analyst material I was, I had a dream which announced that before I became an analyst I had to get the permission of 200 mothers.

Through my prayers to the mother goddess I developed a feeling that she was with me at all times and that she literally was my body. It was a whole new concept to me, the idea that the body is God, and the body therefore is to be worshiped. When I asked the mother who she was, she said:

"I am the basis and the bottom of your life and your beginning. Your body still is mine, as it always was, my gift to you. Love me in your body, and in your body worship me."

I stopped worrying about being vain or narcissistic, and I just gloried in how beautiful my body was. Then came a gentle soothing energy through my body that seemed incompatible with any illness.

Kieffer, my spirit guide, also emphasized the divine nature of the body. "The body," he told me, "is the most important thing. It has been neglected because people do not live within their bodies, but always within their senses and in the outside world. The body is mostly an object they talk about and do research upon. Our sense and our thinking are the least of God and the most of man. But God is in the body.

"When one worships the body and glories in its graceful forms and mysterious functions, the body regains its splendor and tranquility. If we love the forms and the workings of the body and adore it as the god it is, then it will glow with nature's power. It will renew itself and will give back radiantly all the love that comes to it. Even in old age as the body withers, it still is beautiful, and God is there."

9
Where Is Passion Bred?

This thing about the body is so important that I'm going to go right on talking further about it. It's the body that is sick, right? And if you look at it more closely, there is plenty of evidence that the body has received insufficient love and attention. In our culture, despite all the so-called new freedom, the body and especially the sex organs are distinctly off limits in any polite society. We seem to be absolutely fearful of certain spontaneous body functions and secretions and unnameable body parts. Not to mention almost any uncontrolled expression whatsoever. When passion breaks loose, it may happen by benefit of alcohol or cocaine or be a sudden, impulsive, unconnected act while the rest of one, the "proper" part, is momentarily out of commission.

I wrote a chapter in a book on holistic healing intended for medical professionals and for educated lay people. The word "vulva" came into my text and, believe it or not, it was edited out. The reason they deleted it, I guess, was because I didn't speak of it in a clinical way as an impersonal body organ, but was describing it as a cushioned, silky, fleecy place, springy like a tiger's paw, slippery and gorged with blood, inviting my entry. In other words I was talking not as an anatomy professor but as a regular person.

In the circles where I travel—and which I am trying to get away from—this kind of detachment is the rule. What's missing is passion. The absence of passion is like a cultural disease, and it ought to be clear that such neglect and denial of the body cannot be very good for the health of the body. I don't want this to sound like a plea for more pornography. It's just that passion is very much in the body and usually gets generated down near the base of the spine in the region of the genitals. Where it goes from there is up to the individual development of the person. But that's where it starts; and if you want to be a lusty, hearty kind of person who's alive in the body, you have to receive the impetus from that basis and stop habitually tuning it out.

In order to free myself up for this kind of indulgence I had to get a lot more intimate with the goddess whose acquaintance I first made in connection with my chest pains. As I spoke with her further, she became in gradual steps more of a love goddess and less of a mother goddess.

It seemed like a terribly big challenge to me. I had felt those longings all my life, almost like a madness seizing me: to see the female form, to crave the sensuous touch, to sense the strange sensations at the pit of the stomach. How could they be kept alive and not repressed, and yet not take form in some wild psychotic episode that acted out my fantasy? I could not keep all this bottled up and yet expect my body not to suffer. The energies need to flow with all valves open, with limbs loose and free and sphincter muscles relaxed. I could not be creative, I could not be healthy, with all the natural channels blocked.

I talked to the goddess woman, who now was more like a wise oracle. I told her of my crazed unreasoning longing, this time for one Beverly, a real live person. "It can't be all bad," I told her, "because my yearning is full of so much dynamic power. I know I can't act it out, and I'm not going to. But what can I do?"

"Please do not repress it this time," she said. "It could kill you to repress it. Do not say it cannot be. God knows how it should go, and you must take your chances. Direct it, but do not censor it."

So she didn't say yes and she didn't say no. The longing was terribly strong, and I had to struggle within myself with the yes and the no. I wrote in my journal as follows:

"I go on day after day, plodding, worrying, conforming, making no waves, receding into the scenery as if I am nothing. Yet here is Kundalini bottled up inside of me. Here is Mercury. Here is Shakti. I am more than I look to be. Why have I chosen this role, to keep Kundalini in the bottle? Fear. Fear. What is there to fear? Shall I open the bottle and find out? Someday, someday before it is gone forever, we must take the risk. We must live before we die. If it is too much, let us find out."

Then I spoke to the lady within: "Do you want me to open the bottle, to embrace Shakti?"

"I do. Open the bottle. Embrace her. But do not ask me how. Feel life. Feel the energy. Let it stir you. Live the power. Always I have asked you to open, to give, to dare. I do not tell you to hide, to cover up, to be nothing. The power is in your pelvis, at the seat of your spine, in your torso. It stirs your lungs. It is tremendous, unbelievably powerful. Feel it. Love it. Live with it. Do not let it disappear. What a blessing! How great a feeling! You are a vessel containing the great life power. What a peace! What a splendor! Always it is with you. Do not let it go. Carry it. Let it move you. Honor it. Love it. Worship it. Let it be expressed in all you do. It is yours to live with. You do not know how it will express itself, but you know that life is nothing without it."

And as she said these words, I felt the feathers sprouting and the warmth flowing up and down my spine.

As these dialogues with the goddess went forward, I became more and more awakened to the intensity of my desires.

Nothing else seemed more important, as if this held my whole salvation and everything of importance and all else could be quite readily thrown aside—career, reputation, wealth—if only I could have this passionate desire satisfied. I realized that this had been with me always, stirring the most ecstatic, most sublime desires. It appeared to me as the center and meaning of everything. All else was meaningful only as it contained this or symbolized this or became a substitute for this.

It was my longing for the sensuous earth woman, but more than that too, as if it held everything that was the opposite of my life to this point, everything feminine, everything sensuous and emotional, all those things I had left behind in my overemphasis of the masculine and the intellectual. And it seemed that the greatest meaning of being alive was to have a body. Live and enjoy it while we have it. As my lustful fantasies progressed, I saw the inner woman more and more as the embodiment of sensuality and the closeness to her as the way to recover my most neglected functions, those having to do with the sensate world, with the sheer physical intimacy, the pleasure of touch and taste and smell, the urge also to unite erotically with another.

It was the love goddess who exemplified all these qualities. Frequently I spoke with her. "It is I whom you crave," she said to me. "You crave the union of our bodies, yours with mine. I have called you to myself to make you whole, to fill your life with Eros. I am the goddess of love. I, Aphrodite. Do you not remember me? It is you whom I crave. It is I whom you crave. Flesh, warmth, the ardor of desire. You cannot do it only in the mind. You cannot do it only within yourself. You must be man to woman. The goddess is everywhere. Seek her, touch her, clasp her, enter into her. Do you feel Kundalini stirring? The warmth and heat of passion rising up? Feel your body. Be in your body. Base of the spine. The caldron heating."

Kundalini was being aroused. Could I handle it? Could I let it activate my being? Could I give it voice and arms and legs, express it, let it live?

"Oh dear one," I cried, "dear Aphrodite, is it you? Enliven me. Enrich me. Take my being. Inhabit me. Be alive in me. I welcome you at last. I will open up the gates and lay aside my fear. Let me take your power and hold it in my hands. Let it tremble. Move me. Hold me. Let it come."

I saw her undulating, writhing, glowing in the darkness. "Great goddess," I exclaimed, "please live in me forever. Never leave. Now I hold your power within me. Feel it stirring, warmly glowing. You have come, and you are with me, dear Aphrodite, ever young. What is life without you? Empty, rigid, dead and old. Now you radiate and glisten. I have opened now the bottle. You are with me. How you glow. This is power and power abundant. Kundalini, Goddess, wonder. I in awe expand my soul."

It seemed to me while undergoing these experiences that nothing in the world exhilarates the body, so filling it with joyous sensations and glowing vitality as the erotic feelings rising up the spine. Naturally such an arousal of Eros affects the outer relationships also, and it opened me to many temptations, so that one needs to have wisdom about when to say yes and when to say no.

I found that the hours with Aphrodite did have an influence upon my behavior. People of both sexes seemed more attracted to me than had ever happened before. And I did things in a way that was new to me. One day, for instance, in talking to a lady friend whom I had never before touched, without any thought or decision my arm went around her, a totally natural and appropriate act.

I had a dream that I was with a woman. No passionate sexual embrace this time. Our cheeks were together, slowly, carefully touching, brushing lips over cheeks and lightly kissing mouth to mouth.

This was one of the most sensuous experiences of my entire life. And here it was, happening in a dream! Not so much at the genitals as it was all over the body. It was sensuality magnified a hundred times by the "imaginative" element, by being in the lungs and all over the body surfaces as well as at the seat of the spine. Even the slightest touch of lips or fingers or the meeting of eye to eye was more wildly thrilling than the most excessive orgy one might contrive.

Continuing the dream further in my imagination, I spoke to her: "We have climbed the chakras together," I said, "and they are all lighted up."

"It is all I could ever desire," she said. "I have entered all of you. Every inch and every depth and every surface. We meet now face to face. The life power is in the face. It is everywhere. It has lighted up the highest levels. God has penetrated your most conscious being, and the ecstasy is great. God is alive in your eyes and in your ears and in your inward vision. Now God will take us down to the core and center, down into God's own realm where the fountain is. Behold, God is with us, and the power is everywhere."

10
The Image Behind the Symptom

I became aware that every pain, every illness, every symptom has a psychological content that goes with it. This is the symbolic part. This is the way our imagination perceives the illness or the symptom. For example, when I talked to my arthritis pain, my imagination perceived the pain as a kind of demon or god who desired intimacy with me. Presumedly as our intimacy increased, he would be less inclined to torture me with pain.

And then with my chest pain there was all that symbolic content about having my mother's body and the idea that I must love and worship the mother through my body. And on the negative side, there was the thought that my mother was pulling me into the grave after her.

The symbolic content is often difficult to get hold of. Nevertheless it is always there. If we let ourselves wander gently into the symptom, the image is right there. After I was cured of my rheumatoid arthritis, I still had some residual pain and weakness in my left foot. I asked Kieffer about it, explaining that I was doing everything I could, massaging it, exercising it, pushing it to harder usage.

"Well, of course," he said, "you do all those practical things, but the real issue is with the symbols. What about your foot? What image does it raise in your mind? Can you tell me about that?"

"Yes," I replied. "I see an old man hobbling with a cane. He's not troubled very much by the lame foot. He has accepted it, and his attention is on other things."

"What things? What kind of person is he?"

"He's very alive mentally. I suppose you might say he is a deep person, religious maybe, a kind of philosopher. He is like a wise teacher. People come to him because he inspires them and gives them insight."

"So," replied Kieffer, "you see. All *that* is centered in your bad foot. It is really non-essential whether the foot gets better or not. That will take care of itself because it's not really the problem. The problem is that you have been unaware of the interesting old man. So perhaps the foot trouble is there so that you would limp a little, so that you would get a feeling of his presence, even for a time feel a bit like him yourself. His presence will probably change you quite a bit. You see, when you stop cursing the symptoms and get deeper into the images instead, then the healing comes. But the healing never starts at the place of the symptom. Your foot doesn't get better. Maybe later, but not as the first thing. First you have to be healed in your soul.

"The paradox is that the wound, the illness, is also the treasure. The physical misery gets your attention. But then if you go deeper into it, there is much more to it, memories and imagination and worries of what will come. As when you had your chest pains, and all those things came back to you—your mother and her illness, your mystical identification with her. Exactly what you needed, to come back to the mother and feel her love and nurturing. That's where the treasure is, in the psychic images that come with the symptoms. The symptoms open you up. They literally tear you open so that the things you need can flow in."

Then in a few sentences he summed up his view of illness and healing. "When you become ill," he said, "it is as if you have been chosen or elected, not as one to be limited and crippled, but as one to be healed. The disease always carries its own cure and also the cure for your whole personality. If you take it as your own and stay with this new experience, with the pain and the fear, and all the accompanying images, you will be healed to a wholeness far beyond your previous so-called health."

To me at this time the big question was *how*. How, when I am so wracked with pain that I can't possibly sit still and reflect?

""Sure," Kieffer said, "you want to fight it, but perhaps when it gets bad enough, when you can't fight it anymore, you will open up. Then in your desperation you are ready to do anything. Maybe you will throw caution to the winds and go along with whatever happens to be there. It's a life and death struggle, testing your mettle. You've got to be open to be cured. Yet some people will never open up. They just keep their teeth clenched and won't change one iota, and they just let it kill them. That's how afraid they are of the images. And maybe for good reason, because if people are that hard-shelled, maybe it's because those images would drive them into insanity. Perhaps they don't have the personal strength to digest the power that is in the images. So it's going to get them one way or the other, either by death or by insanity. Yet it's a good sign if one is conscious enough to see this dilemma. Then, with such consciousness, there may be enough spiritual power in the person to deal with the images. It's your fate. Better to stand up and face it."

"Well," I said, "I guess I'll have to take the chance. I'll let all the craziness in and hope it doesn't overcome my sanity. Stay with me, Kieffer. I need you."

"What I'm talking about," said Kieffer, "is the big diseases, not just headaches and indigestion and such stuff. These could just be the result of wrong living, and they are easily remedied. I'm talking about the overwhelming things that you can't really blame on the person or on his bad health habits. An outside force comes along with no logic whatsoever and completely wipes you out. It has the power of a religious experience. Then one curses God and asks, "Why me?" as if there ought to be a cause and an effect. As if we did something wrong. Don't feel guilty. Don't blame yourself. Perhaps it's something in your fate. God doesn't punish you. He selects you. He shows you with an almighty power that he is there. He favors you with his attention."

Then he pointed out to me some of the ways I was holding back from letting the images and all their power come through to me.

"There are a lot of things wrong with you," he said, "and you should be worried. You won't walk into your places of fear. You skirt around the edges of things. It is because you are afraid of your own body and your own reactions. You might blush. You might stammer. You might cry. The body won't stay under your control. So you avoid the unpredictable situations—no tears, no sobbing, no runny nose, no blushing or fainting. You see, it always gets back to the body. You're afraid of it. But remember, we already established this: The body is God. The body is something to be worshiped. It's not for you to control. This is the big thing, you and the body. Remember, it's your mother; it's the great goddess. Love her for her great gifts to you. Let her be herself in you."

11
What If I Like the Way I Am?

When people are sick, they want to get well. Period. They don't want to change their personalities or their attitudes or any of their habits. Consider, for instance, the smokers with emphysema who can't stop smoking, the alcoholics with floating livers who can't stop drinking. So if these people can't stop, when cause and effect are so obvious, what can we expect when the causal links are more subtle?

People who are sick with a really dangerous disease will often be willing to submit themselves to non-medical forms of treatment. Usually they will like it better if the "treatment" is something which is done to them, so that they are merely passive participants—massage, soft music, the laying on of hands. Some people will gladly offer themselves for biofeedback or hypnosis. They may even be willing to attend a religious service that calls forth divine healing energies. Or they may be adventurous enough to experience the sweat lodge, the chants and the drums, the spells and incantations of a primitive healing ritual. Any or all of these things might have a wholesome effect, but the healing will be lasting only if such experiences help to launch the person toward a new way of life.

Psychotherapists sometimes explain to a suffering patient that migraine, for instance, is caused by their perfectionism, and if only they would be more easy going and relaxed, the headaches would go away. Or the cancer patient may be informed that her disease comes to "nice" people who never get angry and who take too much of the blame for everything that goes on around them. Then she might be advised to be a little tougher toward others, a little kinder toward herself, and to live more for pleasure and less for duty.

In other words, I am saying that it is possible sometimes to identify the personality that goes with the disease. We can say to the patient with some validity that if he or she could change the ingrained behavior patterns, the illness might quite possibly go away. The trouble is that knowing such facts seems to have little or no effect upon the physical condition of the patient and may, in fact, even make it worse.

The truth is people do not change by being told that they need to change. Even if they agree, they are usually totally unable to bring about a genuine change of attitude and behavior. And if a change is forced out of sheer will power, it is not really a change but only a source of greater stress. The most damaging part of all is the guilt. Most people feel inferior and guilty enough already just for being sick, and to put on another load of guilt, hinting that they caused it all to happen because of their neurotic adjustment, creates the absolutely worst kind of mental atmosphere for healing to occur.

The paradox is that they do need to change their behavior and their mental outlook, but they cannot or will not do this, and to tell them they ought to do something they cannot do makes the whole situation even more insurmountable. Nevertheless, in many cases there is a definite need for a total restructuring of the personality. The need is to become more nearly what nature intended them to be and to let go of all the neurotic baggage loaded upon them through no fault of their own.

When Kieffer spoke about getting at the image behind the symptom, he brought up the importance of sliding into another dimension. It is a way of seeing the disease in its non-physical dimension. It is a look at the "soul" of the disease. But he also cautioned that we shouldn't be too one-sidedly over-eager to get rid of the symptom. The symptom isn't really the problem. It is merely the visible manifestation. The problem is in the total way of thinking and feeling and acting. The symptom is a kind of indicator that something has gone wrong with the total mechanism. Most people ordinarily cannot face such a possibility, the possibility that their whole life and their perceptions of life up to this point have been erroneous. It is hard for them to contemplate the idea of killing off their old self and starting all over from scratch with totally new assumptions. Yet that is just about what needs to be done.

And actually the sickness itself is part of their growth toward this "revolution" in their viewpoint. The sickness assaults them and effectively demands that changes have to be made. Unfortunately there is many and many a case-hardened individual who will not change. Their theme song is "My Way." Their motto is "I like the way I am," even when hardly anyone else can stand the way they are. Yet the more self-blaming people also often cling doggedly to their old ways. To be a re-educator or a psychotherapist is not an easy task. The patients, deep in their bones, hardly ever want to change. And yet deeper in their bones they really do desire change. Deep within is a wistful yearning for reconciliation with a long lost self that they only faintly remember, if at all.

I have found it necessary to go against common sense. It does not work to say to the sick person, "Look at this fact and look at that fact about your sick soul. They have contributed to your illness, and if you want to get better, you will need to change these things." That kind of straightforward sensible approach does nothing except make people worse.

So if someone likes the way he is, I say, "Fine, that's a good start. I'm glad to see some sense of well-being and self-satisfaction. That's what we need."

Also I would tell the person that right within him or her are all the tendencies and all the right feelings and healthy instincts that can rescue them from this slump.

"I'm glad you like the way you are because you'll find even more of yourself to like, and I just predict that it will show you the way to feel even better and to like yourself more than ever."

Obviously the least helpful thing in the world would be to impress patients with more guilt and blame for making themselves the way they are. It is the more buoyant, more harmonious and enlivening feelings that stimulate the healing energies. Certainly not more guilt.

However, we cannot expect such healthful attitudes and wholesome changes to occur just by prescribing them. The goal is to be individuated, to be fertilized, regenerated, transformed, and therefore to be healed of one's ills. We cannot command it to be so or wish it to be so. Nor can we expect to cure the symptom without curing the whole person. The healing process in its true sense, therefore, is individuation. Individuation is a coming home, a kind of rebirth into one's true, authentic and complete self.

The patient, as I have indicated, cannot choose to do this or be instructed to do this. It is not a logical process, not subject to will power or to any reasoned stepwise procedures. It is a miracle of nature. All we can do as therapists is to charm the person into the process. Then, being there, nature leads the way and performs her miracles.

So we are assuming that within each person there is another side to things. There is another person within them. Let's call it the child they used to be. There is also another way of thinking. Let's call it fantasy or imagination, or the world of dreams. If I as a therapist can charm them into entering this world and taking it seriously, they may become interested in it and captivated by it with a deep concentration and a renewed willingness to believe and to be involved in the same kind of complete way they were as children at their play. Then, if they've done that, they've accomplished an important thing. They've let go of their usual serious self-directed ego position with its emphasis on common sense and control and conformity and caution, and they've let the easier, more natural way carry them along with its flow.

If they stay with this fascination, if they let themselves be shaped and renewed by their excursions into the world of imagination, they will no longer be the same person they were before.

12
There Is a Story

When I said that it is the more buoyant, more harmonious and more enlivening feelings that stimulate healing, I hope that this was not misunderstood. Such positive, healthful feelings usually are not there right in the beginning. Nor can we manufacture them out of will power. Nor does it do any good to avoid, to repress or deny all the negative thoughts. Even the guilt. I didn't say get rid of the guilt. I just said don't add more on top of what is already there.

There is one guideline that is more important than any other, and that is truth. We have to be totally and completely truthful with ourselves. So-called positive thinking is a pale, sentimental sort of thing if it is just a covering over of reality. The soul does not thrive on deceit. Truth is the elixir. Truth is the panacea. Truth is the most precious of psychic ingredients, and it is almost a synonym for God.

"Let's face it, Old Man," I had to say to myself. "You have cancer: C.A.N.C.E.R. There is a good chance that you will die before the year is over."

There is always a great tendency toward denial, and we have to know how to get around it, how to get into the reality of the feelings and stop covering them up. When I am in my role as psychotherapist and I have to deal with such a denying person, I do know that if ever they will be able to break through, it is now. Now that the disease has pummeled them and weakened them, perhaps now the distressed child underneath is ready to call for help.

Even when all the therapeutic skills have failed, there are

still dreams. A dream may come, and the dream is like a savior bringing hope, suggesting a way. The dream is the voice of soul. Its function is to get us in line with the journey of the soul. This is the most important thing to do. Remember, we are ill in the first place because we got disconnected from the journey of the soul. We need to get back into the story. This is the story of our life, and the dream comes up to remind us.

"Remember," it says, "this is the story. This is what is happening now, and this is where you should be."

C.G. Jung discovered that dreams have a compensatory function. They bring up what we have left out. They tell the other side. They say, in effect, "This is also true. Do not forget these other big events that are also going on." The dreams urge us toward becoming more complete, more truly and more fully our authentic selves.

They also make us feel good because they are connecting us with long lost friends. It's like a reunion, a coming home. And they bring symbols which are full of power, which have a great appeal and fascination. They have the power to capture our interest much as an exciting suspenseful story book that we can't put down.

Yes, that other side is alluring. It will draw us to another world. And then it weaves a spell around us till we no longer know that world from this. The dreams are as real as life itself. And life is like a dream. Where one lets off and the other begins does not seem to matter.

What is best of all is that it feels good. There is a remarkable loss of tension and a gentle pleasant glow. The story goes on—in our dreams and in the life around us. The ability to suspend our disbelief and to recover the imaginative ability of the child is the greatest advance we can make toward true health.

There is an on-going story and we are in it. It doesn't matter whether it is pleasant or unpleasant. It is only that it is the right story. Then I have found my story, and I know in myself without any shred of doubt that this is where I should be. Then one does not even ask, "Am I happy or am I unhappy?" I just am, and it is right and good that I am and that I am here and doing what I am doing. I have no inkling of where it will go from here, and that does not bring fear, but only excitement and novelty. If I am fully in the story, that is my greatness and my joy. This is the *amor fati* (the love of fate), a condition greatly to be desired.

My fate unfolds. I am a child, and my life is revealed to me. Things happen—strange and new—overcoming me. It is the future unfolding, always fresh and new, always surprising, a fascinating drama that holds me spellbound to my sacred path.

13
There Is a Power

During my illness with rheumatoid arthritis I learned how limited was my mastery of my body. Try as I might, I had no ability to make it well. I did not control the body. I could take no credit for its basic design and function. My body did not really belong to me. The illness began to improve only after I acknowledged my impotence.

Look at it this way. There are a lot of things about ourselves that we do not control. We have to get used to the idea that powers are at work inside of us. They make things happen that we do not want to happen, such as symptoms and diseases. They also for the most part work silently and benevolently, running this miraculous organism without any direction or cooperation from us.

Now, what if it were possible for us to actually cooperate with this tremendous force that inhabits us and controls us? What then?

Let's for the sake of familiarity call the force God because that's what it has always been called. It's already clear from our discussions so far that the life-threatening diseases seem always to have a god or an archetype behind them. These words—god, archetype, symbol, the sacred—are for all practical purposes synonymous. We've been shutting them out, and they want to get in. They break down the doors, forcing their way in, and in so doing cause terrible wounds and disabilities.

Now what one ought to do is to go about developing a relationship with these powers. That is the only solution. All the other possibilities lead either toward death or toward insanity.

The process of cultivating an alliance of some sort is an endeavor that is as old as civilization. It has long been done out of the hope that some kind of covenant or understanding between the sacred and the profane would make things better all the way around. Hence all that long history of rituals, of animal sacrifices, of temples being built, candles burned and billions of rosaries being recited. Perhaps our ancient ancestors knew something that we in our sophistication have forgotten.

A more modern way of accommodating these forces is called Active Imagination. This is the method, already illustrated, by which we meet and converse directly with the divine images. This approach recognizes that God is indeed within us, right inside the body, and that we can feel the God power there in our bodies and can actually communicate with it. This is quite contrary to the more popular idea that God is "out there" somewhere, in heaven or on Mount Olympus, or being omnipotently everywhere, knowing everything and running everything, but not specifically too terribly interested in you and me.

I first got acquainted with this phenomenon of the divine presence within the body by reading about it in *The Perennial Philosophy* by Aldous Huxley. This is a study of the great mystics of all times, and it quotes extensively from their writings. When they have had that experience of the presence, they frequently have reported a strange sensation of heat in the body.

I noted a similar thing when I was in a Quaker work camp as a conscientious objector during World War Two. Sometimes at the camp I attended Quaker meditation meetings. In these meetings one fellow camper while in deep meditation would sometimes be seized by a trembling of his whole body. I never talked to him about this, but I presumed he was having a vivid experience of the presence. I do know that he was by no means an eccentric or a neurotic, in fact he was one of the most respected of the camp members, known for his wisdom, his fairness, his gentleness and stability.

There is a power, no doubt about it. Often when we experience it, it comes in a way that is quite unpleasant. There are dramatic bodily disturbances, such as hyperventilation, tachycardia, high blood pressure, even epilepsy, paralysis and temporary blindness. People wake up from nightmares with their knees shaking and their teeth chattering. There are periods of depression and anguish which have been called "the dark night of the soul." And often, curiously, neither the patient nor his cadre of doctors can furnish any convincing explanation of why such things are.

But here is something we do know: Go deeper into your darkness, whatever it is, and anxiety will change to joy, misery to ecstasy. Remember when I was talking to my pain? When that image formed in my mind of this pain as a divine being, and I felt its presence in every joint of my body? As I spoke to it, a warmth came into me and it radiated through my body. The experience was of a being, an intelligence, not merely an energy. There was also the knowledge that it was aware that I was aware of it. It was like a stream of divine love caressing my crippled body.

This was a revelation that suddenly gave me the whole answer to everything. If only I could learn to recreate this happening. If only I would be able to carry this presence around with me at all times wherever I went. I had read accounts of sudden healing brought about by the laying on of hands where some individuals were able to transmit a healing energy into the body of another, and this energy often brought about astonishing improvement and feelings of well-being, even the cure of conditions which doctors had considered hopeless.

Investigators who have studied such cases have observed that the healing appeared to proceed in the well-known ways that nature heals, by the natural action of antibodies and the normal anabolic functions of the body. The difference is that the healing takes place in a more highly charged way and at a greatly accelerated speed.

Obviously we are on to something. Can we define it? Can we show others how to have the same experience? If ever, if just once, they feel the tingling warmth and know that they have been divinely touched, they cannot help but change the values of their lives. And never thereafter will they cease to yearn for that unique communion.

My own purpose became to cultivate my relationship to this energy so that ideally it would be with me at all times, like an inner companion filling me with well-being, with confidence, and with the feeling of being deeply loved. I felt assured that if I were able to sustain such a condition, my health problems would gradually disappear.

14
More About the Power

I became intoxicated with the idea of power. It was the only thing of any importance at all. Wherever I went, whatever I did, I was always seeking the power. Some life experiences had it and some didn't. And it was a completely individual thing. What was power for me might be nothing at all for someone else. If a person, an object, an activity had no power for me, I was completely bored and I turned away. Life is precious. The power is so life-giving, so sublime, so energizing. Why waste any moment of my short remaining life on anything other than the power now that I have discovered it?

"I'm sorry, Mr. Periwinkle, I cannot spend any more time with you. You just don't have it for me. There is no power."

It's amazing how this attitude simplifies one's existence. It's so easy to recognize and discard the non-essential things. It's like a compass that guides me on my path. It has nothing to do with snobbishness because the thing of power may be the most mundane and unassuming object imaginable. It is simply and solely what awakens the shivers in me.

Those shivers, that electric current that makes the hair of my flesh stand on end, can happen in many ways. Often it comes upon me unawares. Yet by inward turning and by calling to it softly I also have the ability at times to bring it forth. What I wish for is to have it with me daily, continually, to awaken each morning to its presence, to let its embrace envelop me as I turn to sleep. Then it is less sudden in its ecstasies, but ever warmly present, containing me and filling me. Then I know that God is with me, and I am well.

With some people, in some situations, there was power. If for instance there was between me and another a total honesty and a trusting openness, then it happened. Often it happens with a patient in analysis, behind closed doors. We have come together for the very purpose of "soul making." It is absolutely true without question, the motto Jung carved over the entrance to his Bollingen tower: "Whenever two or more come together in My name, I am there." Because we meet for a higher purpose, our souls are awakened and the gods are present.

When I am vulnerable, weakened in my ability to cope, stricken with disease or pain and mindful of approaching death, then I am more attuned to nature. When we are humbled in our littleness, meek and subdued, we are acutely aware of God around us everywhere. And so as ego touches archetype, then paradoxically the sickness makes one well.

The power is everywhere, in all of life. But we are limited in our ability to see it. So we have to look for the special things, the things that are still able to touch us.

Once I found on the beach a lead sinker, the kind used by fishermen. It had a line attached in such a way that it made a pendulum, as perfect a pendulum as one might wish for. And, having found it, I saw it as a divination instrument. It will give a yes or no answer when held over objects according to whether it moves clockwise or counterclockwise. I take it out from time to time when I need to feel its power in my hands or when I wish to seek out the wisdom of the gods.

One day I discovered maggots in my garbage pail. Rather than recoiling with disgust as I had always done before, I marveled at their vibrant energy. I felt like the ancient mariner who, when he had been struck by the splendor of the slimy water snakes, was able at last to pray. Then the winds blew, the ship moved, and hope was reborn.

15
Terror Or Ecstasy?

Why does the power sometimes break in forcibly upon us? Usually, when it comes, it is more than we can contain, much too hot to handle. It comes in a nightmare or in an overpowering fear of the dark or the unknown. Or we see it in whatever disturbing object we project it upon. But not always negative. It can be a vision or a realization, a sudden burst of joy or passion, but always with the feeling of an "other" who has invaded our space.

The more closed we are, the more encased in our little ego world, the more shocking its entry, the more unknown and uncanny. If one is too rigidly closed, it never breaks through to consciousness at all. Then it will strike the body instead, sometimes causing very serious illnesses.

Ideally, when we are in "Tao" or a "state of grace," we will be consciously in harmony with the other powers, and the encounters with them therefore will not be so violent. However, in practice most of us avoid and deny these powers, unless sickness or psychosis breaks down the barriers. Then we face them, and a mighty battle ensues. Either the gods consume and demolish us, body and soul, or else we keep our sanity and are able to enlarge ourselves to include these new realities, and thus we flower into a greater soul.

There is a person I know, Henry, a friend of mine, who had originally been a graduate student in pharmacy. In time he became dissatisfied with the constant memorizing that it entailed and the long lonely hours in the laboratory. It seemed to him to be sterile, boring, and not what he wanted to do with the next 50 years of his life. So one day with a mixture of fear and gladness he switched his whole career to psychology. Then one afternoon he spent a few happy hours with all his new psychology books, and then lay down for a nap.

Then, as he tells it, "I apparently was just entering sleep when suddenly, with a maddening rush of fearful inner intensity, I felt my body vibrating uncontrollably in a violent manner. It was over as suddenly as it began. Perhaps I lost consciousness for a few seconds. I couldn't be certain. I felt extremely weak and was initially afraid to move lest I find that somehow I could not. I recovered completely after a few more moments, however, and immediately speculated about whether it had indeed been a mild epileptic seizure."

After a few weeks there was a similar seizure. He finally went to the student health center to be checked out on the EEG, but no physical cause could be determined.

The frequency of the seizures diminished gradually till they dwindled down to a few times a year. He earned his doctorate in clinical psychology, he married and had children and tried not to think any more about it. He never mentioned it to his young wife, even when she wondered whether he was aware that he sometimes shook a bit in his sleep.

Then late one afternoon when he was in his early thirties, an incredible experience took place. Let him tell it in his own words:

"The seizure suddenly began coming upon me. I was just about to experience the same terrible intensity of its peak when there was a spontaneous shift into a simple but wonderful dream. In the dream I saw my much loved but long dead grandfather sitting on the porch steps waiting for me to come home from work.

" 'Grandfather, you're alive!' I shouted in joy.

"At that very second, it seemed as if the peak terror of the seizure experience was shunted into the joy of seeing grandfather in my dream, and I experienced a wave of ecstasy instead of a mad epileptic panic. At another level of consciousness I was aware of the seemingly accidental union of the two experiences. I made an immediate decision that should the seizure ever return, I would think of my joy at seeing my grandfather and would convert the fearful intensity into ecstasy.

"And lo and behold, it worked! Through my thirties and forties I became quite expert in converting the prodromal signs of a 'subclinical seizure' into the experience of ecstasy. I still told no one about it, but I was quite pleased with myself.

"Some years later, in my late forties, I had the really big experience that taught me humility again. For some time my ecstasy-converted seizures had continued at odd, always unexpected intervals, once or twice a year. Sometimes they were tiny and sometimes moderate, but nothing, it seemed, ever to worry about. That suddenly changed one afternoon when I was seized with a megacharge that began about the middle of my spine and rushed into my brain with such intensity that I was instinctively aware that I could not control it. As it poured into my brain, I was awash in a pure liquid light, brighter than a thousand suns. I felt absolutely paralyzed, certain that I was blinded permanently at the very least. Another second and it seemed as if my brain would shatter.

"Then, through no effort of my own, the intensity began to abate with what seemed to be a very loud hallucinatory rush of sound, like the beating wings of a crowd of birds or bees. And, as the intensity diminished further, the sound became that of heavy bedposts knocking against the wall because my body was vibrating so violently that it was shaking the bed against the wall. But all this must have been a dream because, in fact, there are no solid wood posts nor frame to my bed.

"It took me almost ten minutes after this experience to recover sufficiently to be able to move and to sit up in bed. I then recognized the similarity between this and the spontaneous experience of Kundalini that was reported by Gopi Krishna long ago. I was very shaken and weak, but not as hurt as he was. I also was very ashamed. All these years I had wasted playing with the seizure-ecstasy in what now seemed to be an idiotic manner.

"If I was to survive, I knew I had to strengthen my body in some way. Physical exercise did not seem as appropriate as yoga training. And so for the past few years I have taken meditation training with the Zen people, the Sufis, the Seikhs, and most recently with the branch of Buddhist meditation known as Vipassana. Mostly my meditation is uneventful and seemingly of poor quality. I can just barely sit for 30 minutes, but at least I do it every day. Every year or two a striking seizure comes, and sometimes I manage to have the kind of mystical experience that is typically reported in the books. However, it does not seem that I have sufficient wit to become wise or enlightened.

"A few weeks ago I had a seizure that seemed to turn into an 'out of body experience.' I had been in a light sleep for about 30 minutes when I felt a seizure begin to come upon me. I was elated at the prospect since I had had no such experience for quite a while. But it seemed that my ego consciousness was too strong and too clumsy in reaching for it, and it began to abate. I pulled back, hoping it would return—and return it did. But instead of peaking in a straightforward manner, it seemed to fizzle backward into some other channel. Suddenly I became aware that I had popped upward for a few feet, much like a bean pops out of a pod. I slowly drifted up a few more feet and then realized with despair that my bedroom was so dark that I could not even make out the outline of my sleeping body below. I tried to stay awake, but in a moment or two I felt myself awakening and slipping back into my body."

Henry's experiences supply for us some additional evidence of how physical symptomatology is closely interconnected with one's psyche—with fear, with hope, with pleasure and displeasure. We see also how astonishingly powerful the archetypal energy is. Henry had thought he was able to manipulate the energy as he willed. In welcoming his grandfather from the world of the dead, he was also opening up to the mighty power of the great father god. As he himself suggested, there probably was some amount of hubris in the self-satisfaction over his ability to turn terror into ecstasy. Now he has to wonder if the power is far greater perhaps than he ever imagined.

What are we to make of the "out of body experience"? In this twilight area between body and mind, we do not know clearly and decisively what is really real. And we are not yet prepared to make judgments, to say, "Do it this way and not that way." As if we have a choice. It happens to us. We do not choose. But we may ask, "Is the organism defending itself? Are we not quite ready for the full encounter with the realm of the sacred?" If we leave the body, then the body does not contain the experience, and then the sacred meeting of body and psyche is not accomplished.

When we become sick, it is often because we cannot go forward with a needed development. New growth energy pushes toward consciousness, trying to actualize itself. If we can take it into us and consciously live with it, then there will be a restructuring and a rebirthing of the personality.

A powerful stranger had invaded Henry. How pleasant that he could see it as his beloved grandfather. It shows in Henry an ability to love, an ability to extend the circle of the ego to include more and more of life's experiences. And when the going got tough, he did not retreat, but strove to strengthen himself so that he could grow up to the new experience. If one can grow in the capacity to contain the invader without being completely blown over, there are feelings of contentment and joy, a serene sense of oneness with all life.

At its best, this realization is not just mental but is also a vibrant sensual reality running through the entire body. And seeing it this way, as I do, I am naturally skeptical of the value of "out of body experiences," except perhaps as enriching events along the way, though not the ultimate wonder they are often thought to be.

16
Bleeding at the Mouth

Georgia, who is in her early sixties, has had pyorrhea since age 18. Lately the condition has worsened, and she has sought treatment by a periodontist in order to prevent further bleeding and infection of the gums. She thinks the symptoms are a direct result of the stress she has been going through. "Whenever I am under stress," she says, "the bleeding increases."

The stress arises from a variety of situations. Mostly her own struggle with her own failure. Or, to put it more psychologically, she tends to overcompensate for her inferiority feelings but never is quite able to live up to her compensations. So she fluctuates between overvaluing herself and undervaluing herself. She thinks, for instance, that if she had any gumption she would leave her husband. Yet she feels quite incapable of facing the hazards of life without him at her side.

Their relationship is the typical non-relationship of two estranged people. He does his thing and she does hers. They meet between the bed sheets and across the dinner table, with minimum eye contact and empty platitudes.

His thing is drinking. After six p.m. it is hard to find the person behind the alcoholic haze. He works at a law office, his own firm, and somehow sustains the ability to get through each day, and to bring in enough money for a golf club membership, Georgia's analysis, a beautiful home and two Mercedes. He is very fond of Georgia's body which he follows around with lust in his eye after the first half liter of wine.

Georgia makes efforts toward breaking out of the dreary patterns of her marriage. The efforts inevitably fail, however, because deeper than all her well-intentioned efforts is the fact that she needs him. And she needs him to be alcoholic. His dependency on alcohol assures her that he will not leave her, and yet at the same time she can feel stronger than him and superior to him.

Dissatisfied with her marriage, Georgia has ventured into many areas, managing always someway, despite her talent, energy and intelligence, to fall short of reaching the goal.

Presently she is in a master's degree program, learning to be a marriage counselor. Although she has been a full-time student, she is a year behind schedule because of delays in finishing her thesis. She has spent thousands of hours and written hundreds of pages, but can't get her data together to form a finished thesis.

Nor is it because of a lack of understanding of her subject. She is almost too well versed, with too many thoughts coming at once and too full of the book knowledge she has accumulated, yet not able to use her mountain of knowledge to achieve a tangible goal. She knows what everyone else has said on her subject, but she doesn't yet know her own ideas.

And her gums are bleeding.

She had a dream: She was at a garage where cars are repaired. There was a rather ordinary and inexpensive Chevrolet there. It was one like her husband had almost bought. The manager was talking to her about the car, and she suddenly became aware that her mouth was bloody. She became frantic with the fear that she would lose a lot of blood. She remembered that she had an appointment with the periodontist but she was already late. She ran out hoping to get to her appointment. She ran into some ordinary people on bikes, and they delayed her. Finally she ended up in the house of a young woman who told her how to get to the doctor's office.

The dream and her associations to it brought out a number of things. The stress on the ordinary car and the ordinary people made her aware of her lifelong fear of being ordinary. Her father was ordinary. Her mother was ordinary. She also thought of her husband as quite ordinary. Yet the external image he projected was not at all ordinary. He had been a military officer and was now the head of a respected law firm. He was good looking. He mingled with influential people. And he certainly would not drive an inexpensive Chevrolet.

In the dream, when she sees the cheap car her husband almost settled for, her gums start bleeding, as if that possible downgrading of the family image is her wound, her fear, her complex. Her husband with his drinking and his general unconsciousness could very well be soon reduced to a very ordinary, or even disreputable, figure. Is all the exterior accomplishment just a thin veneer that could easily vanish? Then she would again be the waif with the bleeding mouth.

Her husband's accomplishments are real, and not to be denied. But she is now aware that he is not the hero she once believed him to be. He seems more like a little boy using her as his mother; or he is the father taking care of her as his little girl. She already half knows of this underground arrangement. Yet nevertheless the picture that shows to the world is vitally important to maintain.

Even though much of Georgia's situation and her background are quite ordinary, she herself has a heroic spirit within her and a determination to overcome her deep sense of inferiority. She cannot stand to be treated as less important than she is, for instance, or as only a woman, or as being incompetent or uninformed. She is in reality very well educated and has an enormous knowledge in a great many areas.

It is not advisable to treat this woman with condescension.

Her periodontist, for instance, uses his little old lady manner on her, and it infuriates her. "Did we take our medicine this morning?" he asks her. She's not a doddering old lady who forgets to take her medicine. She is sophisticated and intelligent, much more so than the doctor. Please be careful how you talk to her.

But why so angry? What button has been pushed? There is a complex here that she is beginning to recognize. She talked to me at length about her parents and expressed an immense anger toward her mother. Georgia has a wound in her mouth, a wound in her basic need for mother feeding and nurturing. She talked of the bleeding mouth and the loose teeth as representing her poor grip on the world, the weakness in her ability to bite into things and get a firm hold.

One side of the complex is in her weak teeth that can't bite into anything. The other side is that of the so-called oral-biting stage. She rages at the bad mother who didn't mother her properly. And in her rage, she grinds her teeth. All her life she has ground her teeth.

When she was 10 years old, her parents found her diary. They read it aloud and laughed about it, humiliating her, filling her with rage, but also with a hopelessness as if understanding and support were impossible in this deficient family. She has no positive memories of her parents, no feeling that they ever satisfied any of her legitimate childhood needs.

In addition to these traumas, she also received the common curse of the female child. The role of women was unquestioningly defined as being less capable, less intelligent, most fitted for homemaking and child rearing, and also forever childlike and undeveloped.

She looked into these memories that lay behind the bloody mouth, and it became more clear to her that beneath all her accomplishments, all her possessions, the fine exterior life and the social standing, there were feelings of inferiority and impotence, and feelings of rage at the injustice. She is a person with a bloody mouth, with a terrible wound to her basic sense of security.

Obviously much of her striving has been toward cultivating an impressive persona and accumulating material things as well as knowledge and skills, all for the purpose of dispelling her inner feeling of little worth, to make her worthy of the love and acceptance that should come naturally to every child as its birthright.

Further discussion of her dream and of all the associations and memories it provoked enabled her to see that the mouth wound pervades all of her activities. She sees how in her relationship to her husband she is recreating early family patterns. She sees the conflict that lies behind her failure with her thesis, her fear of setting out on a career. As she gets greater consciousness, the stress and the other symptoms seem to exacerbate. As if her determination to break through into a new freedom also awakens all the latent strength of her resistances, so that now, in this time of transition, the conflict increases and she seems to be getting worse instead of better.

Soul making is not easy. All that immediate material that lies behind the symptoms is difficult and disturbing, oftentimes beyond human endurance. Yet this is it, and this is where we start. We can endure it at all only if we have a vision, only if we have the faith that it leads somewhere. It is the quest for soul that inspires us and enables us to endure danger and hardship. Because somewhere, sometime, we had an experience of soul, and the memory of it will encourage us through thick and thin to keep going.

Yet it is not all turmoil and darkness. We are reclaiming

parts of ourselves, acknowledging that this too is myself. Along with the acceptance of all of ourselves, both good and bad, there is a relaxation and a fullness because now we are more whole. We are more reconciled. We have made a start toward taking into ourselves all that we are. There is a good round wholesome feeling in the fullness and in the wholeness and in the freedom from the tension of the war within ourselves, the hiding from ourselves and from others the truth of what we are. Truth is the panacea. So while we are horrified at the exposures of our hidden shame, we are also instantly lightened and renewed.

Georgia is far from being healed. But she has entered into the images behind the symptom of the bleeding mouth. She is awakening to the lost sad child who needs comfort and support. She is feeling her intense anger at being minimized and neglected. She is aware of her fear and the lack of strength to go forward with her fate. These realizations are a beginning, but they alone do not bring healing. Jung has said that the only true therapy is contact with the symbols, that is, with archetypal images. "The least touch of these contents," Jung said, "brings an experience of the eternal." And it is through their influence that we are "fertilized, inspired, regenerated, and reborn."

Georgia has made herself ready for the entry of the symbols. The confession and exposure of her own darkness and the consequent humbling has emptied her ego of its inflation, has enabled her to see the limits of her power and the dimensions of her need. As the ego recedes from its aggressive domination, a way is opened for the entry of the symbols. Being aware now of her great need, she knows what to ask for. "Ask and you shall receive."

When I last saw Georgia, she reported what was a new experience for her. She had been walking in the woods with her dog, "and," she said, "I suddenly felt together. I knew what it felt like to be my own person. All the guilt was gone, and I felt perfectly at peace with myself. As if everything was all right, nothing to worry about. I could take care of myself. Or perhaps something was taking care of me and everything else."

Georgia has started her soul's journey. She has a belief now that she will find her way into her story and let her heart be drawn into the archetypal drama. She must come to the understanding that the bleeding gums are not the essence of her problem. The problem is soul. The renewal of her body and the progress of her soul will both be assisted by her willing immersion in her fate.

17
Anxiety Can Kill

Richard's father died of a heart attack. His brother died of a heart attack. And Richard in his early fifties also had a heart attack. It was as if he had been waiting for it and expecting it for some 40 years, ever since his father's death. Fortunately he recovered, and he is now in psychotherapy

It appears in retrospect that quite early in life Richard had developed a very poor self-image. He feared that he would never be able to live up to his parents' ambitions for him nor to what his school, his community and his peers expected of him. Hard as such demands are upon most young people, they were doubly hard on him because he was definitely different—more sensitive, more artistic, more conscientious, more easily disturbed by criticism. And on top of all that, in his late teens slowly it dawned upon him that he might be homosexual.

This was a terrifying possibility, particularly in his small-town community. He kept it from everyone including himself, for even the thought of being such a "pervert" was more than he could contain. Consequently his whole adjustment became an elaborate denial of his true nature, of all his seemingly abnormal characteristics including his sexual orientation. Almost everything true and real about himself had to be hidden as he sought to convert himself into what his small-town culture regarded as a normal young American male. He dated girls. He even became engaged—several times. Also, despite his deep inferiority feelings, he made a strenuous effort to excel.

He was a member of the high school varsity basketball team, co-editor of the high school annual, secretary of the senior class. His list of accomplishments appearing under his picture in the school year book was the longest of any member of his class.

His later achievements involved an MBA degree at a prestigious Ivy League university and a position with a nationally known corporation. He became in his forties the president of this corporation at a salary perhaps ten times as great as the most affluent of his high school classmates. All this despite the fact that the corporate business world had very little intrinsic interest for him. It was merely the vehicle for proving his adequacy and his unequivocal masculinity. His more natural interests were in music, literature, psychology and art.

Somehow through all of this he felt like an imposter. He especially felt like an imposter in his marriage, never actually being in love and having no sexual desire for his wife. Their social life, mainly with other executive types and their wives, was boring and uncomfortable. He had nothing in common with these people. And yet it seemed the thing to do. His whole life was a charade, stressful beyond endurance, playing a role that was foreign to his nature.

Even in his college days the stress had been tremendous, and now it was getting worse, probably because he had become more and more deeply imbedded in a life that was totally false and unsupported by his true self.

What he called his "anxiety pains" had begun in high school and recurred spasmodically ever since. These entailed a lump in the throat, tightness in the chest, rapid heart beat, flushed face and high blood pressure. Along with them came the fear that he was going to die, which, of course, further increased the anxiety.

So predictably, at age 53, he had the heart attack he had always been expecting to have. Although there undoubtedly was a hereditary predisposition toward heart disease, his life style must have also contributed to his condition. This view is substantiated by the great reduction in his anxiety symptoms as psychotherapy brought him more in touch with his true self and effected changes in his behavior and life style.

Richard did not retire immediately after his heart attack, though he could well afford to. He stayed on in his conscientious way to get every detail in the proper order. However, the heart attack did at last convince him that he was living a life that was totally unsuitable for one of his temperament. What was he trying to prove? He was now in psychotherapy with me, and he was undoubtedly influenced by my view that a total realignment of his personality was urgently necessary if he was going to survive.

He decided to retire, but this too was stressful at first. Being at home so much, he became more acutely aware of the falsity of his marriage. Also he sometimes impulsively entered a pornographic movie, and he became stirred by the sexual actions of the nude males. Never in his life had he had sexual contact with a man. Yet he yearned for it, and he teased himself with the thought of it. There was no one he could speak to about these yearnings. He didn't know who he was or where he belonged. And he was still very frightened of the possibility of another heart attack.

The angina pains in his throat and in his chest were coming as frequently as ever. He felt sure they had something to do with his inner sense of security and well-being. "A part of my personality is causing it," he said, "and it's telling me I need to take care of something, that things are going in a pessimistic direction, and it's up to me to do something about it. It's a sign to me that my health is deteriorating."

"If there were an emotion behind it," I asked him, "what

would it be?"

"Fear," he said. "Fear of death, of disease, of my vulnerability." And he went on a bit about how he wanted to get away. To live all by himself for four to six months, maybe forever, to do what he likes, to make his own friends. He needed at least to see what it would be like. He'd be lonely perhaps, but he had to find out who he was without other people's ideas distracting him.

"Jane doesn't understand me anymore," he said. "She keeps wanting to get me back to where I was, to do things with her as her spouse. But it isn't me. It's all a lie. She doesn't understand me at all. Just says I'm being selfish. And maybe I am. I don't know. But I just can't do it anymore. There's nothing real between us. I have to get away, but I'm afraid to. Am I being selfish?"

Then a few days later he again had those feelings in his throat and chest, his "heart disease symptoms." This time the tightness in his throat felt like a presence that had come in and inhabited his body. He called her the Witch Lady, and he decided to have a dialogue with her.

RICHARD: Here you come again. How can I get rid of you? I suppose it was because I was enjoying myself today. I met some new people and they liked me and made plans for me to be on their staff as an advisor. People respect me and admire me. Then you come along and grab my throat and make me feel guilty, as if I've done something wrong, threatening me with heart attacks and death.

WITCH LADY: You are wrong if you think I'm being critical of you. I just want you to be absorbed with me once in a while. You are always so excited about those big deals and achievements that are going to make you feel important. Why can't you forget all that stuff? It just keys you up and makes you nervous and tense. I only want to get your attention. If you pay a little attention to me, your life would go a lot better.

RICHARD: I don't want you or anybody else to rule me. I don't want to be an artificial personality. I just want to be myself.

WITCH LADY: But you're still afraid of sickness and death. You don't have the guts to be yourself.

RICHARD: Yes I do. You're helping me get back on track. I have been afraid. I keep procrastinating. I haven't had the guts to be myself, but it's clearing up in my mind. It seems more and more important to live by myself for a period of time. I have to choose between two high risk courses, either continue on as at present or go out on my own.

WITCH LADY: Well, I guess you're the one that has to decide. Maybe for once you'll make your own decision. It is so easy to manipulate you. I can churn you up as if you were buttermilk. You give me so much power over you. The answer is in you. Don't push yourself. Try for once to be your own natural self.

He followed this dialogue with some fantasies of what he would do if he had his own apartment and his own life style. He would get a place with a small garden, with books and a stereo, a place where he could walk on the beach, be close enough to see his therapist weekly, attend a men's discussion group, and just follow his instincts wherever they might lead him. Then he wondered, would he get lonely at times? Would he miss having someone like Jane who was committed to him? Would he be able to develop new relationships? Would some things of value slip away from him, his family and his friends? There was no guarantee that he would find a better life, but the alternative of staying stagnant in his present circumstances seemed to be more and more impossible.

Then he had a dream:

"I was in a university environment talking with a young student who was wearing a soft leather mask covering his face. There were goggles over the eyes and a filter for breathing. It seemed very natural that he should be wearing this mask. The young man had a strong personality and spoke with conviction. A portion of his eye could be seen from the side of the goggles. His eye under the goggles seemed very strong and alive.

"I was thinking that I should like to have a similar mask. It furnished a look that I liked, in a fashion sense, sort of like Darth Vader.

"The young man finished talking to me, and he left. Later he appeared without the mask, and he seemed rather ordinary."

Richard associated to the dream. He thought of the mask as one's persona, the face one shows to the world or the role one plays in order to function in the world. It somewhat hides the person underneath, but it nevertheless projects an image of masculinity, sensuality and mystery, all of which he admired. It was a kind of life adaptation that Richard could feel good about. It perhaps overcompensated for his indecisiveness that the Witch Lady had talked about. It balanced out his habitually pleasant agreeable side with some tough substance from the shadow side. Hence it was stronger and more real. To carry out his radical plans, he may have to be willing to be the bad guy.

"I've worn a mask for many years," Richard said. "It has cut me off from a direct connection to life and to others. I would like to have this kind of persona, if I could pull it off, and if I could still also know who my real self was underneath and not just spend my whole effort wondering if my persona was effective, without the fear I would be found out for what I am. But what am I anyway? That's what I want to know."

He then associated to the eye that was under the goggles. He thought of the eye as the lamp of the body, remembering a passage from "The Sermon on the Mount":

"The lamp of the body is the eye. If your eyes are sound, you will have light for your whole body; if the eyes are bad, your whole body will be in darkness. If then the only light you have is darkness, the darkness is doubly dark."

And he read further:

"No servant can be the slave of two masters; for either he will hate the first and love the second, or he will be devoted to the first and think nothing of the second. You cannot serve God and money.

"Therefore I bid you put away anxious thoughts about food and drink to keep you alive, and clothes to cover your body. Surely life is more than food, the body more than clothes. Look at the birds of the air: They do not sow and reap and store in barns. . . ."

As he read these lines to me, he broke into uncontrollable tears. And I was deeply affected also. Although I was well acquainted with "The Sermon on the Mount," the part about the eye being the lamp of the body was totally unfamiliar to me. But it exactly stated the whole thesis of my work on healing: "If your eyes are sound, you will have light for your whole body. If the eyes are bad, your whole body will be in darkness."

How clear it is in that quotation that the most central function most directly affecting all the others is the truth and the clarity of vision, the function of deeper consciousness, the soul function. It was for me a moment of synchronicity wherein the symbol that touched Richard's most sensitive hot spot also touched mine.

A few days later Richard dreamed that he was returning to his graduate school of business. He was going to enroll again for classes. It was as if he had an urge to go back to that period of his life and do it right this time. Perhaps he could learn to be a businessman without losing his soul, to adapt to the modern commercial world yet not totally blot out and obscure his true self.

There was in the dream an object called a lamp, but more complex than a lamp and which also included a telephone. When he plugged it in, it heated up and exploded in flames. He asked for help, and a technical person brought another of these lamps and helped him set it up. A part of the lamp instrument was an enormous cock that he held between his legs. It was artificial and overly large, but very realistic. His helper, the technician, remarked that in Jamaica, where these cocks are made, men's cocks must be really huge. The technician then began getting all the equipment together in the right arrangement. Meanwhile Richard was enjoying the feeling of the enormous cock between his legs, and he stroked it sensuously. Another part of the lamp apparatus was a workman's leather belt with tools attached. Among the tools was also a supply of condoms, and it appeared that the whole belt arrangement was a sexual kit of some sort, and Richard was now ready for sex, as if sexual proficiency were an art or craft at which one could become a competent professional workman.

Richard called this his "Big Cock Dream." Later in the dream he was talking to his home-town minister back in Alabama, telling him about the lamp and the big cock. Unfortunately this minister is of the old repressive school, and was highly embarrassed by the linking together of Christian ideas and big cocks. At this moment in the dream, Richard took his own blood pressure and found that it had risen to an alarming degree.

Here we see how in the course of one week, by attention to his inner life, Richard has brought to his awareness some of the psychological content that has been imbedded in his symptoms. His blood pressure, for instance, is heightened by the conflict between the morality of his home-town minister and the new consciousness arising within him. He is finding "instruments," concepts, adjustment mechanisms, to strengthen and reinforce his masculine modes of adaptation. He has an image of the eye as the lamp that lights the body. He is beginning to feel the possibility of bringing the sexual and creative energy into his physical body and into his concrete life adjustment. And he is seeing too that his angina pains in the throat and chest are associated with a witch woman and that they may also be an equivalent or substitute for his deep anguish and thinly covered sobbing that locates in the same areas. He has also acknowledged that he has been trying to serve two masters, and this is another conflict that requires solution.

Now with all this psychological content to his problems, he can perhaps deal with the anxiety as a psychic phenomenon, and he will not need to see it wholly as a physical symptom that he can get rid of only by physical measures, such as rest, diet and medicine.

The truth is that when anxiety is repressed, it is pushed down into the body and becomes physical tension which in turn produces further symptoms and real physical disease. As the conflicts and the anxieties are seen in their psychic reality as worrisome memories, as fearful expectations, as danger of loss of soul, and as one looks at the dreams and the fantasies that illustrate the nature of the psychic disturbance, then one gets closer to the true unvarnished facts of oneself. Momentarily as we look at the full horror of our psychic condition, we may become more anxious, but, because we are taking on the necessary suffering of the soul, the body relaxes. And because we are no longer running away, the truth seems not as abominable as we had feared, so that there follows before too long a deep feeling of peace. There is no longer anything more to fight against once we have accepted everything we are.

Richard has now come to believe that in following his own way he is not being selfish, but is earnestly trying to be true to his nature and to balance his inner truth with the reality of the life around him. Now when the chest pains come, as he explained, "Sometimes the pain is like God, as if someone is telling me to watch out, saying, 'You can go at any time. Watch out! You could drop dead.' He won't let me forget it. It makes me want to be sure I don't make any mistakes. I don't want to be on the wrong side of God. Even in my prayers I now include the words, 'I accept my death as part of God's plan.' "

By daily facing the reality of death, death has lost its sting. It is now a reality, part of the whole of life, not the cause of unexpected anxiety attacks.

If psychotherapy is to be a healing influence, it will heal not only the emotional complexes and the psychoneuroses, but it will also simultaneously heal the body. It has to be so, because body is not separate from mind. What affects one affects the other. If people suffer from physical disease and assure us that they have no anxiety, no disturbing dreams, no images or fantasies that go along with their symptoms, then we have to assume that on that particular level they are quite unconscious. Then as psychotherapists it is our job to facilitate the emergence of the psychic material, to help them see how the physical disease is viewed by the soul.

If we can ever get through the thick layers of armored resistance, something very tender or volatile or convulsive is touched. And when that gets touched there is also a definite physical reaction. For example, Richard began sobbing convulsively when he read about the eye as the lamp of the body and the idea of serving two masters. His blood pressure elevated when his new-found "lamp, big cock, sex equipment" came up against the attitudes of his home-town minister.

Our place of greatest vulnerability is also in the same region as are our most severe physical symptoms. This place of greatest vulnerability is also a holy place, a place of healing and a place of miracle. Those hot spots seem to be connected at first to our guilts, our fears, our personal conflicts and unpleasant memories. But just pursue them a little more, go deeper, and behind them are the archetypal images, the power of the gods.

Richard's experience was typical and not unusual. By going into the psychological content behind his illness, he came to his personal struggles, and behind them very quickly came the more profound archetypal events, in his case the comfort of tears and the words of Jesus, the divine healer. We serve our patients best when we are able to bring them again and again to that place where the mundane ego and the sacred archetype meet and touch.

18
All Over the Skin

Melanie had suffered from skin rashes for a good part of her life, and they had become especially unbearable within the last 5 years. Although she had been in analysis much of this time and had achieved some significant growth, the skin trouble persisted. She had some logical ideas of how and why, but unfortunately the reasoning mind cannot make symptoms go away just because it knows how they got there.

Finally the symptoms were dominating her waking thoughts and keeping her awake half the night. They became the principal subject of her journal writings, and in her desperation she started talking directly to the rash itself.

As she wrote in her journal:

"The rash is really stinging now. It is up my back and more intense in its itching. What is going on? Obviously I'm not living my own life. I thought I had worked things out, but not so. I am jittery and nervous and feel as if a tremendous force is raging under my skin. Sometimes I think it is the Self wanting embodiment. Or something is demanding that I get out of this environment."

Then she began speaking directly to the skin rash.

MELANIE: Rash, now you have my complete attention! You burn and rage under my skin. I am aflame, and I don't know your meaning.

RASH: I have been with you forever and have only been manifesting in this outrageous manner for the last 5 years. It's about time you paid heed to my assaults.

MELANIE: Yes, you are assaulting me, and I don't understand your purpose.

RASH: You have failed to talk to me. I demand your full
attention. Then all else will fall into place.

MELANIE: I thought I had done that.

RASH: You try this and that to alleviate my fire, but that
isn't the point. You must enter into my fire and endure my fire.
Then and only then can we be together as one, under the skin,
deeper than skin.

MELANIE: I feel that you are inside me, flaming forth,
wanting to erupt into my life. And I want that too, but I don't
quite understand what you have in mind. And also I cannot let
you burst forth. Your power could overtake me, and even
those around me. I fear your power. You can destroy me.

RASH: I can and I will if I don't get your undivided attention.

MELANIE: You have it. You have it. I am here to bring
you into my life as much as I can.

RASH: You have denied me too long, and I am raging like
a fire out of control.

MELANIE: Yes, I believe you. I cannot make you disappear. Not even with ointments and creams, not even with al-
lergy medicine. I have a fantasy of running through the streets
with my body afire, aflame, a living incendiary. You are pursuing me, and I cannot escape your fire. You are agonizingly attached to me much as a fire shirt.

RASH: Yes, I am pursuing you, and I am a shirt of flame
burning myself into your very soul. You have to bow down to
me now.

The next day the rash was as uncomfortable as ever, but
she was beginning to think of it differently, and she also had

become engrossed in the dialogue and was curious to take it further. Besides, with all the pain and itching she couldn't very well think of anything else. The dialogue resumed:

MELANIE: Well, Rash, you certainly haven't left me alone. You are back again in full force, demanding all my attention.

RASH: I do demand it. You have to bow down to me now.

MELANIE: I know you want my undivided attention, and you do have it. You have been with me for long periods. I recognize you first in terms of being rash, acting rashly. All my life I've been pulled to do things impulsively or with wishes for my own aggrandizement. Now that I realize my rashness, I tend to question my every thought and move, asking, "Am I being grandiose?" I have given you much thought in the past 5 years. I have not fully understood you, but now I am trying to understand.

RASH: You cannot understand me with your mind alone. You have to accept me into your life. I am under your skin. You can no longer ignore me!

MELANIE: Yes, I understand.

RASH: You have been trying to get rid of me! That can no longer be. I am your fate, and you have to love me, both in my benign state and in my more malignant states.

MELANIE: Yes, but it is difficult when you are plaguing me and bedeviling me.

RASH: You will bow down to me. You will love me no matter whether I am nice or ugly. I am with you to the very end. You have put me off for so long, and I will no longer be put off!

MELANIE: Again, I understand, and I admit that I do love you. I am yours, and you are mine. We are bedfellows together. We are in the same skin.

The next day Melanie wrote the following in her journal:

"Something has happened. Suddenly around 5:30 I felt together, whole. I felt self-confidence. I felt integrated and in charge of my life. Was it because of the active imagination? I hope and pray that I can continue to feel this way and to be a help to the people I work with, letting your love flow through me."

But then in a few days the rash came back again in all its glory, and she wrote as follows:

MELANIE: I am trying to tolerate your searing, flaming, burning, itching assault upon my being. You have my undivided attention. I scratch compulsively. I have to be careful which clothes I wear so that I don't aid and abet your flaming activity that seems like a brush fire upon my skin, raging at all times.

RASH: Now I see that I have your attention. You omitted one descriptive phrase. I am the fire-bath of transformation. You have to endure the fingers of flame as they dart over your body searing the nerve endings of your skin. I am burning deep into your soul. You will never forget me. You are fated to endure my flames. Just as I have manifested in the rashness of your thinking and doing and moving, I now manifest in the purification of those activities, purifying your soul until all that remains is pure and wholesome. I am your shirt of fire to remind you of your greed and lust for power which is no longer acceptable in my sight.

MELANIE: Somehow your statements make the suffering more endurable.

RASH: It's about time.

MELANIE: Now you sound like my father. He said something like that before he died when we all sat around the dinner table and became emotional at the blessing. I felt put down by that remark. It was not the father being joyous at the son's returning home. You are stern and unforgiving, I feel, with a remark like that.

RASH: I see your point, but you have to admit that it is about time.

MELANIE: Yes, I realize it's time, long past due for such an experience. You are both hell fire and the transforming essence.

That evening she wrote again in her journal, expressing some of the deep feelings her dialogues had evoked.

"What is attempting to break through? What rages out of control? What wants to erupt into life? I want to be free! I want to live my own life! I want to wake up when I want to, get up when I want to. I want to be myself. Is this rash representing the spirit? Is it something that wants to manifest in my life which I fear will take me over? I am a living death without spirit. Spirit gives meaning to life. I need to let it into my life. It is the essence of life, the life force coursing through my veins."

And then she continued the dialogue.

MELANIE: And still you are there. Still you have my un-divided attention. My flesh breaks out in stinging sensations as if in spontaneous outbursts of flame, first here and now there. My hands are constantly busy trying to extinguish your malicious little darts.

RASH: Yes, I truly have you in my grip, and I want to live in the same skin as you.

MELANIE: I accept that, but I don't know how to consider

it. I say yes, come on in, but you keep on needling me with your darts of flame which cause eruptions of hot lava. It is deliciously painful and exceedingly diabolical of you. Are you trying to build a fire under me? Are you trying to urge me to some creativity? Is that your goal?

RASH: I have told you that you cannot avoid me. I am the fire of creation. I am the fire of damnation. It is only your use of me that determines what I am.

MELANIE: I believe that, but when I look around me to see what it is that will lead me forth into a creative venture with you, I do not see a line of direction. How can I use your creative flame? In my usual work and activities? Or is there more that you want me to do?

RASH: I want creative expression. I want to come into the fulness of your life in a creative manner. I have the energy for it; you have to supply the method and the hands.

As a result of these confrontations with the power behind the rash, Melanie greatly deepened her understanding of things that had eluded her for years. She had previously misunderstood the nettle rash and the hives and the welts, thinking them to be prods and goads that were pushing her, perhaps out of guilt, to more activity, more attainments and more awards.

In fact, to some degree she perhaps continues this misinterpretation, thinking that she has to "do" something "creative" rather than merely developing a more loving harmony with the "fire god" and letting its magic have a home within her. Then she will know what to do and need not figure it out.

This case is another good illustration of the depth of emotional experience that is evoked by attending to the images that lie behind the symptoms, and how by a deep and sincere interaction with these images, dramatic and rapid transformations take place. It is also a very good example of the experience of the power.

The psyche manifests itself physically. It wants to be part of our bodies and part of our concrete empirical existence. That fire which produced the tortuous skin condition is the same fire that has been called "the presence." It is that same sprouting of the feathers of the soul. As such it can bring gladness, ecstasy, health, and the overflowing of love. And we see again that the greatest treasure comes out of the most despised and secret places, from that which is the basest and the most humiliating.

Melanie's previous work with her skin problem had been too intellectual. She gained information, she learned theories and she constructed probable scenarios of how it all started. Yet all these interesting speculations actually accomplished very little. That is because the body reasons in its own way, following patterns that were laid down even before we knew how to talk, before memory, before consciousness, certainly before any ability to think. We cannot think our way out of psychosomatic illness, nor out of any of our unconscious complexes.

Experience is the catalyst that can shake up existing patterns and bring about a change. Not knowledge, not thinking, but experience. The kind of experience that is crucial in such transformations is the experience of the transcendent—the power, the presence. The written dialogues with inner figures, or any other kinds of encounters with them, are very real happenings with very real consequences. These events are invariably more profound in their effects than the most vivid of concrete outer experiences.

If we will commune inwardly, preferably by writing, with devotion and deep concentration, before long the gift will come. Then in a breathtaking encounter we will meet the miraculous one. Changes then are automatic. We are no longer the same person. We have become one who has met the great power and who has lived to remember it.

What is interesting about a skin rash is that it may very well be a sprouting of the feathers of a soul that has somehow gone wrong. It is as if the god got into us and around us and all over the skin, but we didn't give it the right greeting. We were so alienated from the god power, and so scared of it, that we had all our armor up against it, and it had somehow to blast its way into our consciousness. One way or another the power, by God, is going to get through.

19

The Problem or the Power?

"What can I do for you? Tell me why you are here. What is your problem?"

Questions like this are the typical first remarks of the psychotherapist upon meeting a new client. There follows then an examination of the problem, probing deeper and deeper into it, as if that problem and its solution were the goals we seek. Yet, necessary as the problem solving may be, it is not exactly in itself a healing process.

One might, in fact, actually get sicker and sicker by reenacting every last memory scene of abuse and humiliation and despair. Unless these sickening experiences can be reassimilated into a stronger and healthier ego, the illness may feed upon itself and fix its symptoms more immovably.

Something new needs to be introduced, something that will turn things around and bring a healing energy. Usually we count upon the personality of the therapist to be the intervening factor. The therapist makes two where there was one, and that brings a new viewpoint, an outside observer, some objectivity. But the most beneficial intervention is in the personality of the therapist. If he or she is a person in harmony, one who is with the larger power, then the therapist's presence alone is healing. It brings the patient closer to the soul self, to the thoughts, images and fantasies of the unconscious. These are things of power, and the power flows into us like a healing elixir. The wonder of the analytical hour is that it can cause this to happen, even to hardened characters who have never had such an experience before.

The important question is not "What is your problem?" but "Where is the power, the creativity, the healing energy?" It is not possible for therapists to mediate the power of the greater unconscious if they themselves have not experienced it.

There is something very special about the analytical experience. It is a unique kind of meeting whose purpose, whether articulated or not, is a holy one, having to do with the meaning of one's life; and behind such a question always lurks the mystery of that which we cannot see. When we come to analysis, we must eventually face the ultimate questions, because it turns out that they are necessary in solving the lesser question for which we thought we came. If the therapist has the appropriate awe, then the patient too will sense that this is "soul work," and then the healing gods will come.

The problems and the power are often strangely interwoven. Those knotty complexes where we are so guarded and so sensitive are the hot spots. They are the nuclei where the energy is locked up. Press that button and the tears flow. Behind the symptoms are complexes—tears, fears, anger and guilt beyond believing. There is in the complex, in fact, more power than seems to be logically explainable. The truth is that the complex is like a soft spot in our armor where the blessed ones can enter—as well as the monsters of the deep.

Jung has observed that every complex has an archetypal core, so that once we enter the area of the complex, we are walking in a very direct route right toward the gods. It is almost a question of which came first. Do we have this complex because it is our inborn fate to have this specific archetype on our back? Or did our life experience with a critical, unloving mother, for instance, make for an open wound through which the archetypal mother made her entrance?

It is important to be aware of the two levels of a neurotic

complex. Stay forever on the level of the guilt and the shame and all the personal misfortunes of your life history, and you are as lost as ever. The power is there, still locked up in the complex and its symptoms. But if the archetypal power is felt and faced and brought within the scope of our imagining, then the individual sufferer is transformed beyond belief. Then there is a miraculous reawakening of human life, a rejuvenation of self esteem. One knows at last that a creator lives within. Then one can say, "I am not alone, for lo, a power is in me, and I am of it." Then out of one's belly shall flow the "rivers of living water."

These are the kinds of results that various churches are promising to us, but why then do so few of their members obtain them? The religious teachers tell us to believe. However, we cannot think ourselves into belief nor obtain belief by will power. Belief comes from experience. It happens to us, and then we know. Only then can we believe. A psychotherapy oriented toward the power of the archetypes can mediate experiences that bring opportunities for communion with the power.

The living water with its healing power is ours only insofar as we get on to the archetypal core of our problems. How can the god powers enter us and work together with us if we deny their existence, if we will not relax from that philosophic rigidity that does not let the rivers flow?

It is not a linear process. You do not find the god in a stepwise way, from square one to square twelve. It's not just sin, confession and redemption, not merely forcing yourself to crawl again through the unsavory muck of long ago.

Yes, you do have to review your past life, but not just to count it all out on your list of sins to do penance for. You need to be reunited with your whole self, both dark and light. Reclaiming the soul in its totality is like looking into the eyes of

God and finding there a chaotic chasm of darkness but also some glimmer of hope.

It is dreary and demeaning to feel again the loss, the depression, the fear and the spiteful feelings. Who wants to grunt and sweat through that stuff all over again? Yet embedded with it is the power of the archetypes. Curiously, as we go into the disturbing places, we are not only disturbed but also uplifted because the archetypal power has been touched. We feel braver and more powerful because the "Great One" is with us. It is not unusual, therefore, that people seem to be getting worse as they are getting better. Now, filled with the energy of the archetype, they are at last strong enough to claim everything that they are, both the dark and the light. This gives a sense of fullness and peace, as if God can now enter because they are simply what they are, open to what is, no longer hiding behind pretenses.

Obviously then, it is most important that we ask where the power is. If we don't have some friendly access to the power, we can't even look at our problem. We're suffering too much already. A little more guilt about the "problem" is often enough to push some people over the brink.

Psychotherapy today is at the same kind of crossroad that exists in religion. Is religion a big list of sins, or is it a joyful reunion with God? This conflict has been dramatically emphasized by Matthew Fox, a Roman Catholic priest who has been officially silenced by the Catholic Church as "dangerous and deviant" and who has been forbidden to teach, preach or lecture.

Father Fox calls his viewpoint creative spirituality. "It is," he says, "the opposite of fundamentalism. It's about trust: trusting nature, including our own human nature, our dreams, our bodies and our imaginations. It believes that passion, Eros and ecstasy are blessings and not curses. It emphasizes creativity rather than obedience, the aesthetic rather than the ascetic. And, above all, it is about cosmology, about resetting the human agenda within the context of the cosmos rather than in the man-made world we've been living in since the Enlightenment." (Interview with Matthew Fox, *Psychology Today,* June 1989)

Fox is very appreciative of the psychology of C.G. Jung and other psychologists who move toward a more spiritual direction. He believes that what is wounded in us is the divine child, the true Self. The most useful healing measures are imagination and creativity. We need rituals and prayers that open our heart to our pain and to the awe, the wonder, the mystery, and the glory

Open to the power!

20

Why Not Change the Plot?

It ought to be clear by now that the state of the soul has a big effect upon the health of the body. The body reflects the psyche. If your soul-self is wholesome and rich with healing symbols, the health of the soul shines forth in the body.

Every illness has a mental or spiritual aspect to it. It is not, of course, "all in the mind," but certainly the mind is somehow in the illness because there is always, if we will look and find it, an image, a fantasy, a story, that goes with the illness.

The question naturally arises: Which came first? Does the illness cause the fantasy? Or does the fantasy cause the illness? If they are interdependent, then perhaps some new input from either direction will bring a change. Alleviate the illness, and perhaps the fantasy life will become "healthier." Change the plot of the fantasy, and the illness will go away. Or perhaps they don't even cause each other at all. Maybe they are all one and the same thing right from the beginning. The symptoms and the fantasies are merely different ways of observing the same elephant. It is you who are different, or your vantage point in looking at the thing, whether you see the ears of the elephant or his trunk, perceiving it sometimes with the inner eye of imagination and at other times through the pain receptors of your body.

At any rate, your soul-self is comprised of the total thing— body, mind, symptom, fear, love, hurt, expectation, dream and fantasy. Mind-body chaos occurs when all these facets of ourselves are not smoothly articulated. Many things can go wrong, such as bad environmental conditions or unsatisfied physical and emotional needs. But the biggest chaos producer is the willful human ego. Human beings have free will and with it the ability to deny and repress and to overrule the bidding of their instincts. And do they ever!

The ego is the eye of consciousness and it has the ability to see and to understand. In a healthy personality the eye expands and sees more and more of the truth of its reality, and in so doing it also forms a relationship with its larger self. Spiritual growth is a process of the ego becoming more inclusive, of incorporating into the ego more of the soul-self. Remember, the eye is the lamp of the body. The more clearly the eye sees all of reality, illuminating one's own darkness and also the face of God, the more our consciousness is like a lamp that lights the body with healing power.

We have to get under the ego and into the unconscious because that's where nine-tenths of the soul is. If that unconscious soul is sick and deranged, it has to be purified.

So let's say you tune into the inner drama. Let's say the plots and subplots you find there are real horrors. Can you change the plot? Can you, in effect, alter your fate? The answer is yes, and the answer is no. Your fate is your fate. You can't change the path of the planets in their course. But you can change yourself so that you are cooperating with your fate instead of fighting it. The tension, the neurosis, the diseases come from being in opposition to your fate. Stop fighting the story. Get into it. Enhance it. Assist it. Make it manifest in your daily behavior. Be an actor in the drama. Add some new ingredients and everything starts changing.

When the body doesn't heal itself, healing procedures are used, forms of intervention. They are founded on the hope that you or the doctor or someone will do something to your sick self that will help it get better a lot faster than just lying there and doing nothing at all.

Theoretically we can intervene from any direction, body or mind. We can alter the environment, find a new friend or lover, change the body chemistry, remove infected body parts. We can read books, listen to music, pray to the gods or cuddle our pet cat. We can also probe the unconscious, letting the dreams and visions and fantasies affect us, and we can in turn try to have an effect upon them.

It is important to note that there is a correspondence between body and psyche. They live in and of each other and what happens to one is mirrored in the other. And quite possibly there is no difference at all. They are both inter-contained and identical one with the other. In our place and in our time, for some reason, the body is overemphasized as if that is real while the soul is non-substantial and therefore non-existent, a product of the imagination or the dream life.

But dreams are real. Imagination is real. They have real effects. They are the causes behind world literature and art and music. In fact all the significant accomplishments of mankind started as insubstantial ideas. The dream patterns within us, the fantasy plots, seem in all probability as if they were the actual cause of many diseases, crimes and serious accidents. A skilled dream interpreter can see these impending dangers in a person's dreams.

Dreams and fantasies are scientific data. They tell as much and in most cases even more about a person than does urine analysis, blood pressure or x-rays. Those fantasy themes that exist in the unconscious are psychic patterns out of which the physical structure develops as well as the concrete behavior.

It has been said that if you are not conscious of your fantasies, they will become your fate. That is because behavior is formed out of the inner fantasy life. And if you are not conscious of the fantasy, it is acted out automatically. It will break through, possibly in a harmful way. However, being conscious of the fantasy, one can chose how and when to live it out. There is the example of William Shakespeare whose fantasy world was full to overflowing with murder, intrigue, with incest, with pathological ambition and revenge. Had he not written his famous plays and thereby consciously expressed these impulses, he might have become the most dangerous of acting-out psychopaths or the most broken of invalids.

The inner psychic patterns, the dreams and the fantasies, have tremendous power. They have the power to kill us or to heal us. When the inner story becomes morbid and unhealthful, we are in for trouble, including the weakening of the immune system and the vulnerability to disease.

It is positively uncanny what happens when people take their dreams seriously and when they attempt with their best efforts to comprehend their dreams, to cooperate with them, to interact with the dream symbols. They open up and become an instrument through which the dream speaks. Healing is promoted by writing dialogues with dream characters, by meditating upon the symbols so that their power comes through to consciousness, by carefully drawing each part of a dream image, by molding it in clay, by acting it out in a dance, by doing research to further amplify the symbols so that their deeper meaning can penetrate into consciousness.

As you follow further with your dream story, you will see a progression. The things that other characters are doing in dreams, you may be doing in subsequent dreams. And the things you do in your dream life you will start doing in your actual behavior. Thus the potential you is being actualized. With a cooperative attitude toward your fate, you will consciously assist the process. If in your dream you are writing a poem, do it. However crudely, start being the poet that you are. Or, if your dreams suggest it, start speaking spontaneously to strangers, start drawing pictures, start making speeches. Make your destiny manifest. Help your whole self to live. It is there already. With your conscious collaboration, it will begin to take a positive and a creative form.

Out of this devoted kind of activity, perceptible and often dramatic changes take place. The story changes because a new influence has come to bear upon it. You too have changed. You have changed in your thinking and feeling, in your behavior and your appearance. Without the response of the ego toward the dreams, they tend to remain forever on the same static themes. However, with the subject's participation, the story moves forward, the dreams become more enriching, more inspiring . The soul is purified. And the body also. You begin to understand those famous words of Sir Gallahad: "My strength is as the strength of ten because my heart is pure."

A pure heart, remember, doesn't mean that you are a pure person. God save us from pure people. A pure heart is a good heart, an honest heart. It means that you have stopped hiding. It means you have stopped pretending to be pure, but have actually become pure by acknowledging your impurities. Confession is good for the soul. Everything that is needed for the soul's salvation, for the healing of body and mind, is already present within us.

21
And After That the Dark

Then up ahead among the things to come is death.

D.E.A.T.H.

One of the serious conditions that older people often have is death anxiety. This is a real killer, a self-fulfilling prophecy. Paradoxically those who want to live well have to learn to die well. You have to know that when the bell tolls, it tolls for thee. When the saints coming marching in, they are calling us to death, even though they also bring a richer life.

One of the most jovial, most humorous, outgoing and buoyant personalities I have ever encountered is Joe Wheelwright, a Jungian analyst from San Francisco who studied under Jung. He told me that ever since he was 35 years old not a day has gone by that he hasn't thought of his own death.

Some time ago I had a dream that I was required to dig my own grave, but for some reason I kept putting it off.

Obviously it was important for me to give more thought to my death and to become more ready for the final days. Being somewhat of a practical mind, I got in touch with a lawyer and drew up a living trust, and I also tried harder than ever to get my soul in order.

Once a person becomes 65 or 70, if not before, there is considerable interest in longevity. We never seem to be quite ready to die. Maybe later but not yet please. It's hard to imagine not being around anymore. How could there even be a world if I weren't here to see it? I didn't exist before, that is true, but now that I am, how can I ever not be? This whole question of being, of body-hood and soul-hood, is a tremendous unsolvable mystery. Yet the thought of death and the preparation for death are very important because they put our lives in truer perspective.

Our little time within this body is soon over, but life in its larger sense goes on. The knowledge of our rapidly approaching death makes us more aware of that other realm where dwell the saints and the archetypes. When we are no longer afraid of death, we also are unafraid of the archetypes, and their power comes marching into our lives

If the miracle of healing I've been talking about really worked, shouldn't we keep on healing ourselves and live forever? Not really. The person who resists death when it is time for death is not healing himself. He's making himself more neurotic and is making for himself a very unpleasant agonizing death. There is a way to die. It doesn't matter when you die so much as how you die. Not by what means, but whether or not you are altogether in one piece, psychologically speaking. I remember frequently those words of Kieffer: "The object of healing is not to stay alive. The object of healing is to become more whole. Death is the final healing."

Now that I have become an advocate of healing, I'm inclined to feel like a fraud as my body ages. They're going to look at me and they're going to say, "Heal yourself Old Man. If your teachings are so great, why aren't you out there climbing trees or something?"

In my weaker moments I worry about this. But it is the ego that worries, with its concern for image and reputation, with its ambition and greed for things of the world. It is not shameful to be failing in health. The only real cause for shame is in losing touch with the soul-self.

The body ages. The immune system is not what it used to be. Let us acknowledge the truth of what we are. But let us be sensitive, very sensitive to the movements of the soul. Stay with the story, so that even in our infirmity we are living what we are. We are fully in the story. We are blessed and happy because in our soul we are healed.

Joseph Campbell advises that we seek our bliss. It is blissful to live our fate. And although it is hard for many to imagine, when we have achieved the *amor fati* and we know that the power is with us, dying is not the worst thing in the world. The time comes for God to swallow us up. We surrender the last ounce of our personal power, and we accept the embrace of the Lady of the Lake.

The dream told me that, like mostly everyone else, I put off the fact of death. I do not prepare for it. In my zeal for health and for healing I overlook that non-reversible fact. I am growing older. We cannot go just with those parts of the story that are pleasing to us. However, just because we feel a little tinge of death, there is no point either to start thinking, "Oh, oh, here it comes. It's all over now."

Part of us may want to let go and just give up. But there is still life energy, and perhaps the closeness of death may even give that remaining life energy a very special quality. At any rate I personally am resolving not to die before my time. I will stay with that life that is in me, and I will live it out. But when it is time to die, then I shall die willingly.

I have watched movies of a tiger stalking a herd of deer, then singling one out and moving in on it for the kill. The deer uses all its strength and speed to stay alive. But when it is finally overpowered and the teeth sink into its throat, the deer yields, almost blissfully it seems, as it embraces death.

The more we are with soul, the less identified we are with the ego. We know our center then to be a larger stream of life transcending ego and going on beyond our death. The soul is somehow in union with this larger being. And as I align myself more with soul and less with ego, the soul's story becomes my story. Then I cannot grieve unduly for the ego. It is like a candle that has had its hour and now must flicker and go out.

Yet now that I have so convincingly taken all the sting out of death, I must come back again to the truth, the whole truth. Inevitably there is a sadness that goes with the awareness of death's approach. It is the sadness of parting. It is also the sadness of not having lived enough.

If parting is such sweet sorrow, death is the most sorrowful of all but possibly also the sweetest of all. It is not just the goodbyes to spouse and lover and friends, but going away from everything, all the things we loved to do, but can do no more, all the things we wanted to do but never got around to. It would be a false bravado to deny the great sorrow of death. From the side of the ego, which is about to be extinguished, death is sad, is eerie, is terrifying. It is nevertheless an adventure, an adventure we fear to face, but the contemplation of which can lift our lives to greater levels of meaning.

Yet, even if I can be truly composed and fully ready for this great transition, there is a sadness for those who love me, and I grieve for their grieving. I am deeply pained by the pain they shall feel. The broken bonds. What once was, no longer is—the touch, the looks, the goings in and out together. Meaningful things done habitually, without a thought of their doing, are now gone forever and deeply missed.

As death approaches and the ego weakens, the unconscious leaks through and before long we are almost immersed in the divine. God, as Meister Eckhart envisioned Him, is "a great underground river," and as we are gently, gradually borne upon its waters, we are supremely content and fully healed.

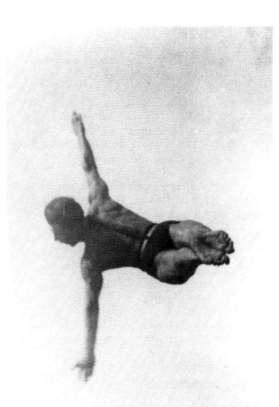

I leave this world as naked as I came,
but an unseen garment holds me
that I hope shall follow to another—
Al Kreinheder, 1913-1990

Studies in Jungian Psychology
by Jungian Analysts

Sewn Paperbacks

New, recent and choice:

Prices and payment (check or money order) in $U.S. (in Canada, $Cdn)
Add Postage/Handling: 1-2 books, $2; 3-4 books, $4; 5-8 books, $7
Write for complete free Catalogue

INNER CITY BOOKS
Box 1271, Station Q, Toronto, Canada M4T 2P4